The Tinnitus Handbook
A Self-Help Guide

by

Bill Habets

United Research Publishers

Preface

This book was originally published in Britain, where a considerable amount of research has been conducted on the causes and treatments of tinnitus. Throughout the book you will come across reference to information sources in Britain. Please don't overlook these useful information sources simply because they come from abroad. It is simple to write to these reference sources and receive valuable information. Check with your local post office to find out the amount of postage required. It's normally just a little more than U.S. postage--and it takes only a few days to be delivered.

Chapter 12 is devoted entirely to U.S. information sources. Most of these sources provide information on natural and alternative treatment sources. One of the information sources is the American Tinnitus Association. It is highly recommended that you contact the Association and avail yourself of the vast resources it provides, especially its quarterly newsletter.

Lowell Housner
Publisher

Foreword

Tinnitus is a very common disorder estimated to affect something like about one in ten of all adults in this country. Despite this high rate of prevalence, only comparatively little research is currently being funded into finding out how tinnitus can be alleviated. Part of the reason for this are the severe budget restrictions affecting the National Health Service as a whole; another reason, generally left unstated, is that there are currently few avenues left open to scientific investigation that are likely to yield major results in the very near future. Nevertheless, research does go on and while no one is predicting any dramatic breakthrough soon, there is a steady accumulation of greater understanding of what causes tinnitus, how it may be prevented, and—perhaps most importantly—how its symptoms can be alleviated by a wide range of therapies.

In the meantime, many a tinnitus sufferer, after having gone through the whole gamut of what the professionals can offer, is eventually faced with the conclusion that his condition hasn't been cured and essentially remains unchanged. That, however, does not mean that there is not a great deal that can be done to minimize both the symptoms of tinnitus and their impact, just that this help will not necessarily be coming from the expected medical sources, but rather from other approaches, these including many simple "self-help" techniques.

As many a tinnitus sufferer will gladly testify, planning and executing your own self-help program is often an excellent way to bring tinnitus under control. Naturally, it is important that before you embark on such a course you should first have all the medical tests and investigations necessary to exclude the possibility that your tinnitus is caused by some other underlying disorder or that it can indeed be cured by medical intervention.

Because what you can do yourself to reduce your tinnitus—or the extent it affects you—is so often the key to making the disorder fade into lesser significance, a large part of this book has been devoted to providing recommendations and suggestions for self-help techniques that have helped many others in the past, and it is my hope that these can also help you.

However, as you read on, please bear two most important points in mind:

Firstly, a book like this one cannot be—nor is it intended to be—in any way a substitute for professional medical advice. Readers are, therefore, earnestly urged to always consult their own doctor before trying out any kind of therapy not prescribed by medically-qualified professionals, starting a new diet, or engaging in what for them is a new form of physical exercise. Only your own doctor—or consultant—can help you decide what may or may not be helpful or appropriate in the specific circumstances of your own case.

Secondly, although the information offered in this book is based upon the views of doctors, specialists and other health professionals, these experts are by no means always in total agreement about many aspect of tinnitus. This means that there are dissenting opinions in many areas and whenever that has been the case I've tried to provide a balanced view of all sides of a particular argument.

Finally, I'd like to say "thank you" to all those who have given so generously of their time and expertise during my research. While they are too many to mention individually, to each and every one of them, my sincere and appreciative thanks.

Bill Habets

CONTENTS

Chapter 1
What is Tinnitus?

It's not all that easy to come up with a totally satis-
factory definition of tinnitus because almost invariably there will be some exceptions to almost
anything you might state categorically to describe
it. To illustrate this point, there is even some confusion about whether "tinnitus" is a disorder in its
own right or merely a label that conveniently identifies a number of broadly similar symptoms.

For example, the authors of one standard
medical dictionary plainly saw tinnitus primarily as
a symptom when they defined it as "any noise (buzzing, ringing, etc.) in the ear." That definition is fine
as far as it goes, but totally ignores the fact that for
many sufferers tinnitus is seen as a disorder or a
condition that is the cause of their symptoms.

It follows from this that the word tinnitus, depending upon the context within which it is used,
can have a curious dual meaning, so at times possibly denoting two quite different things:

1) Tinnitus can simply mean, as suggested
   by the dictionary quoted above, "a noise
   heard in the ear," or

2) The word can describe a disorder of hearing whose main symptom is that the sufferer experiences sounds for which there is no matching source in the environment. But, as we shall see later, this already broad definition still isn't quite wide enough because it doesn't include that form of tinnitus in which the sufferer hears non-environmental sounds that in fact have origins in his or her own body. What's more, *this* definition also fails to include those situations where the tinnitus noises are doubtlessly the symptoms of some other clearly defined disorder. It also needs to be pointed out that the noises of tinnitus are by no means always heard in the ear; many sufferers describe their symptoms as "sensing noises" somewhere in their head.

While it would be useful if there were one word to denote tinnitus as a symptom and another to indicate it as disorder, that unfortunately isn't the case. This means that throughout this book the word tinnitus will of necessity be used as it has been traditionally, to either denote the symptom of hearing noises in the ear or, in its broader sense, as a general label for a disorder or, if you prefer, an ailment or complaint.

Incidentally, for most people affected by tinnitus, there is little doubt as to exactly what the word means to them: it's the disorder, condition, ailment, call it what you like, that afflicts them, and the symptoms this produces usually are simply described by them as "noises" rather than tinnitus.

A Very Ancient Problem

The term tinnitus is derived from the Latin word *tinnire*, this meaning a ringing or tinkling sound.

Because many forms of tinnitus are the result of overexposure to very loud high noise levels over lengthy periods, it is assumed by some that the complaint is a malady of modern times and perhaps didn't exist in earlier days when life was allegedly simpler and probably less noisy. It's a nice theory, but one that's not borne out by the facts as references to tinnitus are to be found in the earliest medical writings dating back to the dawning of civilization in early Mesopotamia and Egypt. In more recent times, tinnitus is frequently mentioned in the medical literature of the day, suggesting that it was just as common a complaint then as it is now.

It is hard to say whether tinnitus is on the increase, although there is plenty of evidence to suggest that there are more recorded cases of it nowadays than ever before, this leaving open the question as to just how many instances of tinnitus might have gone unrecorded in the recent past. Most experts, however, agree that it is likely that more people than ever before have tinnitus today or are at greater risk of eventually developing it, this increase being brought about by several quite different factors, including:

◆ Many cases of tinnitus can be traced back to previous exposure to sounds that were loud enough to cause hearing loss, this loss usually taking place almost imperceptibly over many years, if not decades. While modern technology has brought us the benefits of an endless variety of home entertainment in the form of television, tapes, records and videos, it has also enabled us to listen to these at volume levels high enough to ultimately damage hearing. What's more, for many, listening to very loud music is not just an occasional pastime, but something they choose to be exposed to for many hours everyday, as exemplified by the popularity of the ubiquitous Walkman and similar devices.

◆ There is little doubt that, mainly because of increased road traffic, our towns and cities have generally become noisier places, the cumulative effect of this noise pollution taking a toll on the hearing of the inhabitants. There is also some evidence to suggest that tinnitus stemming from working or having previously worked in noisy environments may be on the increase despite various regulations meant to control noise levels in the workplace,

◆ Even medical advances in other fields may have contributed to increasing the risk of tinnitus. Several drugs used to treat quite ordinary conditions have been found to be able to trigger the problem in susceptible people.

◆ Another reason why a larger percentage of the population may nowadays have tinnitus is because, on the average, we live longer than our ancestors. A very common form of tinnitus is the one that is associated with a kind of hearing loss that occurs mainly as part of the ageing process. As more people live longer, greater numbers reach the age when tinnitus is likely to become noticeable.

Incidence and Prevalence

When considering how widespread tinnitus is, there are two separate aspects take into account: its *prevalence* and *incidence*, two words that are sometime carelessly used as meaning the same thing, but which have quite different definitions:

◆ **Prevalence**—also known as the *prevalence rate*—is a measurement based on the number of people affected by the condition in a given population.

◆ **Incidence**—also known as the *incidence rate* or *inception rate*—is a measurement, usually obtained by statistical methods, of the number of *new* episodes of an illness or disorder arising in a given population over a specific period of time. Incidence is most often expressed as so many people affected or episodes of the disorder per 1000 individuals at risk. In tinnitus, of course, there will almost invariably only be one episode per individual affected, unlike other ailments, such as influenza which someone may have more than once within the time period being studied.

While there is unanimous agreement amongst experts that tinnitus is extremely common. There is some discrepancy between the statistics from various sources, but the following figures are generally accepted as reflecting most accurately the magnitude of the problem:

◆ The British Tinnitus Association says that "more than four million British adults have tinnitus, as do a large number of children, almost certainly from birth." While no exact figures are available for the number of children affected, one estimate extrapolated from other statistics puts this as high as possibly a million.

◆ A fairly old study—but one with an interesting point of reference—was carried out by random sampling between 1957 and 1959: nearly 40 percent of those older than 55 years had a history of tinnitus as did more than 20 percent of people aged between 18 and 24. However, these very high figures need to be discounted somewhat because they also include instances where the tinnitus lasted only a very short time and didn't recur thereafter.

◆ A more recent research project, also based on random sampling, by the Institute of Hearing suggested that a more realistic prevalence figure was 17 percent of the UK population, including only those cases where the symptoms were constant or present most of the time and excluding those where the noises were only heard temporarily. Incidentally, the same study also found that people in manual occupations were twice as likely to have tinnitus than those doing non-manual work.

◆ The British Tinnitus Association has calculated that, on the average, "every day some 200 people in the UK experience the onset of permanent noises in their heads heard only by themselves."

Even more revealing of the massive effect that tinnitus has on the everyday lives of those afflicted by it are figures showing *how much* it affects them. In a recently published document, the British Tinnitus Association said that of the four-million plus adult sufferers in the United Kingdom:

◆ More than 200,000 of them experienced symptoms so severe that they were unable to lead a normal life.

◆ About 437,000 were afflicted to the extent that they described the quality of their life as being "severely affected."

◆ More than 655,00 said that they were "severely annoyed" by their tinnitus.

◆ Nearly 1.1 million described their tinnitus as "moderately annoying."

The sufferers falling into the four categories above add up to about 2.5 million, leaving a further 1.5 million adult sufferers with tinnitus who say their symptoms cause them relatively little discomfort, annoyance or interference with daily life.

While statistics are undoubtedly open to interpretation or liable to slight error, there is little doubt that tinnitus is a health problem of massive proportions, affecting perhaps as much as a quarter of the population at one time or another. To make matters worse, tinnitus is often a medically incurable condition; most sufferers have to find a way to live with it, as confirmed by this comment from The British Tinnitus Association: "For the great majority of sufferers, the most they can hope for is relief from the consequences of tinnitus. . . . Proper counselling can teach people to adjust to the condition. But personal management of it has to be learned, often with difficulty and most hospitals are poorly equipped to teach these techniques."

That last quote may appear to suggest a bleak outlook for most tinnitus sufferers, but in fact that isn't necessarily the case. Hundreds of thousands of sufferers—some of them with very severe tinnitus—have found ways of overcoming or minimizing their problem, using methods and techniques like those described in later chapters of this book.

Chapter 2
How Hearing Works

To fully understand the various things that can go wrong with our hearing—including, of course, the possible development of tinnitus—it's useful to first of all understand how human hearing works. Incidentally, it's worth noting that the original function of the ear in creatures lower down the evolutionary ladder wasn't to perceive sounds but instead to control the proper positioning of the body in three-dimensional space. In fact, the maintaining of balance is still the ear's principal function—even its only function—in many species.

In humans, hearing—which can be roughly defined as the receiving and the interpretation of sounds—is an extremely complex process, involving many different aspects. Although the ears are generally viewed as the organs of hearing, the correct recognition of sounds also requires the proper functioning of the auditory pathway—a series of stages through which nerve impulses are eventually transmitted to the brain.

However, to begin at the beginning, let us start by looking at the ear, which in all higher vertebrates (but also in some more primitive animals) consists of three main parts:

1) The outer ear (also known as the *external* ear). This consists not only of what is commonly called the ear (the flap of skin and cartilage on the side of the head), but also includes the tube that leads from the ear to the eardrum;

2) The middle ear (also known as the *tympanum* or the *tympanic cavity*) is an irregularly shaped air-filled cavity located beyond the eardrum where the vibrations received by the eardrum are transmitted via a series of small bones to the oval window which lies at the start of the inner ear;

3) The inner ear (also known as the internal ear or sometimes referred to as the *labyrinth*). As suggested by the last of these names, this part of the ear is made up of a convoluted system of cavities and ducts, most of which are concerned with maintaining balance, but it also contains a large central cavity—the *cochlea*—

where the received sound impulses are processed and transformed into signals that stimulate the nerves of hearing.

Let us look at these various parts in greater detail.

The Outer Ear

There are two parts to the outer ear: the *auricle* or *pinna* (that is the visible part which lies outside the head and which is that part of the body most commonly understood as being described by the word "ear" when used generally); and the *external auditory meatus*, a tube that leads through the temporal bone of the skull to the eardrum.

The auricle serves but little—if any—auditory purpose in man as it's too small to make a great contribution to the efficiency of the collection of sound. Neither can the human auricle be moved to an extent sufficient to help pinpoint where a sound may be originating. While the human ear can be slightly moved through the action of three muscles (the *anterior*, *superior* and *posterior auricular* muscles), most people are unaware of this possibility although a few have developed the ability of move their ears, this, however, is usually a party trick rather than a way of heightening hearing.

In contrast to man, many animals—especially those with larger or funnel-shaped auricles—can exert considerable muscular force on their auricles and so considerably improve their ability to both collect and locate the source of sounds. Incidentally, there is little doubt that man—or his Darwinian ancestors—once had greater conscious muscular control of his ears and used this as part of his survival skills. In many ways, it's a great shame that this ability was more or less lost as we climbed the evolutionary ladder because even now you can easily test how greatly a mobile ear can heighten sound awareness by gently manipulating the shape of your ears so that they are directed at what would otherwise be quite a faint sound source.

Inside the auricle lies a hollow—called the *concha*—and it is in the deepest part of this that the external auditory meatus begins. This meatus—in anatomy, the word means a passage or opening—is usually about an inch long and slightly curved in shape, with approximately the first third of it cartilaginous and the remaining two thirds bony.

The external auditory meatus is lined throughout by skin, which contains both sebaceous and ceruminous glands, the latter believed to be sweat glands that are modified so that instead of secreting sweat they produce *cerumen*, the medical name for ear wax. An excessive production and/or accumulation of ear wax can, of course, be responsible for both deafness and tinnitus, something that will be dealt with in greater detail in Chapter 5.

The Middle Ear

At the innermost end of the outer ear's external auditory canal lies the ear drum, a membrane made of skin and very thin collagen fibres that, unless damaged, completely seals off the outer ear from the middle ear. A muscle—the tensor tympani—that runs from the ear drum to the wall of the middle ear keeps the ear drum under tension, so making it more responsive to sound waves.

A chain of very small bones—called the *auditory ossicles*—are located in the middle ear and their job is to transmit and magnify the vibrations perceived by the ear drum to the oval window which lies at the opposite end of the middle ear. There are three ossicles, the first two acting as levers upon the next one in the chain and the last one acting directly upon the opening to the inner ear:

◆ The first ossicle is the hammer (the *malleus*). It is attached to the upper part of the ear drum and therefore responds to vibrations induced there by sound waves, transmitting and amplifying these to the next ossicle.

◆ In the middle of the chain is the anvil (the *incus*). This receives vibrations from the hammer, and amplifies these once more, before transmitting them further along the line.

◆ Last in the chain is the stirrup (the *stapes*), its nonmedical name stemming from its shape which does indeed resemble that of a stirrup. The innermost end of the stirrup lies directly upon the oval window, the small opening in the skull that marks the entrance to the inner ear. The stirrup receives vibrations from the anvil and amplifies these as it transmits them to the oval window.

As you can see, the ossicles provide three separate stages at which the sound vibrations are magnified, the amount of amplification becoming greater and greater as the vibrations proceed along the chain.

However, apart from that produced by the lever effect of the ossicles, further amplification also takes place within the middle ear because vibrations captured by the ear drum—which has a relatively large surface, this averaging 85 square millimeters—are eventually received by the oval window whose average surface is only 3.2 square millimeters. This difference in surface areas creates amplification because when the same amount of force is applied to a smaller surface, its intensity is increased, and this is exactly what happens with the pressure created by sound. One way of understanding this effect is by thinking of a given amount of rain falling down. If all of the rain is spread over a large surface—like a lawn—then each square foot of it will only receive a small amount. However, should all of the same quantity of rain be concentrated within a single square foot that area would indeed be subjected to a veritable deluge.

The two amplification processes in the middle ear—the lever action of the ossicles plus that resulting from the different sizes of the surfaces of the ear drum and the oval window—combine to bring about a massive total amount of amplification, the vibrations reaching the inner ear being between 20 and 25 times more powerful than they were when originally received by the ear drum. Because the effect of this magnification can in fact become too intense when the sound level is extremely high, there is also a mechanism through which it can be automatically damped down and this consists of a muscle—the *stapedial* muscle—that reduces the build up of oscillations in the ossicles by pulling the stirrup somewhat away from the oval window. Unfortunately, this damping down effect depends on reflex action and this reacts too slowly to allow people to avoid the damage that may be caused by very sudden and extremely loud noises, such as gunfire.

Other Aspects of the Middle Ear

As has been noted briefly, the middle ear—like the outer ear—is an air-filled cavity. Naturally, so that the ear drum responds only to air pressure caused by sound waves, it is vital that the air pressure within both the inner and the outer ears be the same. Should the pressures not be equal, the ear drum would become artificially distended inward or outward, depending upon whether the air pressure in the middle ear was higher or lower than that created by atmospheric pressure in the outer ear. This equalization of pressure is achieved through very narrow conduits—the *Eustachian tubes*—one of which connects each inner ear to the *pharynx*, this being the tube that extends from the top of the esophagus to the base of the skull and links into the mouth and the nasal cavity. Most of the time, the Eustachian tubes are closed, but they open—in response to involuntary muscular action—when you swallow or yawn. If the pressure in the middle ear at that moment is not identical to atmospheric pressure, then either more air will be admitted to or some will released from the middle ear through these tubes.

Incidentally, it is to deliberately open these tubes that you're often advised to swallow when you're going up rapidly in an aircraft, a time when the atmospheric pressure may be changing quickly depending on how effective the plane's pressurization is. Swallowing under those circumstances will often be marked by a brief "popping" noise in the ears, this being the result of the ear drums responding to air pressure equalization in the middle ear.

Of course, it would seem that the whole problem of matching the air pressure in the middle ear to that of atmospheric pressure would never have arisen had Mother Nature chosen to design the Eustachian tubes so that they were permanently open. There is, however, a very good reason why the tubes are closed most of the time as this reduces the risk of infection affecting the middle ear. This natural fail-safe mechanism can nevertheless be defeated when you blow your nose too violently as this can drive infected material through the Eustachian tubes into the middle ear, possibly resulting in earache or temporarily diminished hearing.

It also needs to be noted that the middle ear provides another important function as it transforms the sound vibrations captured by the ear drum—which, of course, are vibrations occurring in air—into vibrations which are better suited for being transmitted in fluid, the inner ear lying at the other side of the oval window being a fluid filled cavity. Fluid offers a different kind of resistance to the transmission of vibrations than air and this is also one of the reasons why the signals received by the ear drum have to be amplified before they reach the inner ear.

The Inner Ear

On the other side of the oval window lies the inner ear. It is filled with a special fluid called *perilymph* and contains a number of cavities, most of which are concerned with balance (about which more later), but also one—the *cochlea*—where sound vibrations are transformed into impulses which can travel along the nerves to the brain.

The cochlea is a tube within which lie three more tubes. Overall, the cochlea is spiral-shaped, looking rather like a snail's shell or about two and a half turns of a slightly unwound clock spring. The widest part of the cochlea lies near and just below the oval window. Just below that the cochlea is also linked to another window—the round window— that lies between the middle and the inner ear.

The three tubes within the cochlea are:

1) The *scala vestibuli*, also called the *vestibular canal*. This is open to the perilymph of the inner ear.

2) The *scala tympany*, also called the *tympanic canal*. This tube also contains perilymph and links to the round window. The scala vestibuli and the scala tympany are in fact connected by a very small opening—the helicotrema—at the very end of the cochlea, but the size of this opening is so minute that it greatly restricts the amount of perilymph that can flow through it.

3) Sandwiched between these two tubes is the third one, the *cochlear duct* (also called the *scala media*), which is filled with a different fluid—*endolymph*—and contains the *organ of Corti* (also known as the *spiral organ*), a very complex

structure that converts sound signals into nerve impulses that are transmitted via the cochlear nerve to the brain.

The cochlea marks an important stage in the process of hearing because it is here that sounds that hitherto had been vibrations, transmitted through the air, via resonating bones or membranes, or through fluid, are metamorphosed into nerve impulses that can be sent to and recognized by the brain.

Broadly speaking, this is how the sounds are changed from one form into the other:

 Vibrations resulting from the action of the stapes on the oval window are transmitted via the perilymph to the scala vestibuli of the cochlea.

 The vibrations affect the pressure in both the scala vestibuli and the scala tympani. Naturally, these changes in pressure also affect the cochlear duct as it lies between the other two scalas.

 As already mentioned, within the cochlear duct is the organ of Corti and this, in part, consists of a continuous membrane—the *basilar membrane*—within which are embedded some 30,000 sensory cells from which protrude very thin hairs. The upper ends of these hairs are embedded in another membrane, the *tectorial membrane*.

◆ As the cochlear duct becomes distorted in response to altering pressures in the surrounding scalas, this distortion also affects the tectorial membrane, causing it to exert a tugging action on the hair cells. The stimulus created by this pulling action then triggers the hair cells into setting off nervous impulses which are then transmitted by nerve fibres to eventually reach the brain.

Maintaining Balance

As already mentioned earlier, the inner ear also contains other cavities whose correct functioning, although not directly connected directly with hearing, can also become affected when there is inner ear infection. In certain instances, hearing problems will also be accompanied by disturbances in the sense of balance—this combination of symptoms, of course, being a pointer strongly suggesting that the origin of disorder is likely to be somewhere in the inner ear. For that reason, it is worth taking a brief look at these other organs, which include:

♦ Three semicircular canals—one of which lies more or less horizontally, and two of which are placed vertically with their planes at 90 degrees to each other. These three structures can be said to represent two adjoining sides and the floor of a cube. Each of these canals is about 15mm long and lies within ducts in the bone of the skull. At the end of each canal lies a somewhat wider area— the *ampulla*—that contains sensory cells which detect movements in the fluid within the canals and then translate this information into nervous impulses.

♦ The *utriculus*—also called the *utricle*— is an endolymph-filled membranous sac that contains a sensory macula that lies more or less horizontally and whose hairs respond to gravity and translate this data into nervous impulses that are sent to the brain, providing the latter with information about how the head is currently positioned.

◆ Similar to but much smaller than the utriculus is the *sacculus*—also known as the *saccule*—which also contains a sensory macula, but one that is positioned more or less vertically, that also responds to gravity and provides the brain with information about the position of the head. There is, however, some doubt about the exact role of the sacculus in humans, some experts believing that it may not play a large role in controlling balance, but may instead be partly involved in hearing, especially in the recognition of sounds of very low frequencies.

This is how these five separate, but cross-linked, organs work in harmony to control both body balance and posture:

◆ The three semicircular canals—acting together like a trio of builders' levels— provide the brain with the information it needs to maintain the body's overall balance, this being achieved through setting off reflex actions in various muscles to place the body in the currently desired position.

◆ On the other hand, the utriculus—aided to some extent by the sacculus—provides the brain with the information it needs to maintain posture.

Naturally, the brain also receives information about balance and posture from other sources, notably from the eyes and feedback from various muscles, and all of this additional data is amalgamated with that which is coming from the inner ear cavities. Dizziness, poor balance, deficient coordination are all problems that can arise when there is a discord between the information coming from different sources, as can happen through disease or malfunctioning of one or more of the organs involved or when seemingly conflicting information is received, such as for example during a ride on a helter-skelter.

In a Nutshell

To sum up the above, this is what happens in the ear during the process of hearing:

1) The sound impulses—which are transmitted in the air as vibrations—are received by the outer ear, the auricle serving as a not too efficient funnel that

helps direct the vibrations into the external auditory meatus.

2) At the end of the external auditory meatus lies the ear drum and the sound impulses cause this membrane to vibrate.

3) On the inner side of the ear drum are the ossicles which together act as chain along which the vibrations are amplified before being delivered to the oval window that separates the middle ear from the inner ear.

4) In the inner ear, the vibrations transmitted to the oval window from the ossicles are then transmitted via a fluid to the cochlea where the vibrations are transformed into nerve impulses.

The Vestibulocochlear Nerve

The sensory impulses generated in the inner ear are carried to the brain along the *vestibulocochlear nerve*. This is the eighth of 12 pairs of cranial nerves and is also known as the *auditory nerve* or *acoustic nerve*, and in medical texts is often indicated by the Roman numeral for eight, as "VIII."

The vestibulocochlear nerve has two branches:

1) The *cochlear nerve* is the nerve of hearing as it carries the impulses originating in the cochlea.

2) The *vestibular nerve* carries the impulses from the semicircular canals, utricles and saccules, that is information about balance, posture, and movement.

The auditory pathways connecting the ears to the brain also have a number of "stations" along the way where nervous impulses are further processed. There are also interconnections between various corresponding stations in the left and the right pathways which allow for the comparison of information collected by the left and right ear, this comparison being part of the process through which the brain determines from which direction a particular sound came.

What Can Go Wrong

Even from this simplified description of the hearing process, it's obvious that difficulties in hearing may be caused by a problem anywhere along its line of transmission. Things that can go wrong and impair hearing, either temporarily or permanently, include:

◆ In the outer ear, the channel may become blocked by wax, this physical obstruction stopping the sound waves from reaching the ear drum.

◆ The ear drum can be damaged and therefore unable to correctly receive the vibrations.

◆ Ossicles can also become damaged or fail to work properly, so reducing the degree of amplification their lever actions normally produce.

◆ Various diseases—discussed in Chapter 5—can interfere with or interrupt the transmission of sound vibrations.

◆ Additionally, any of the three parts of the ear can be become infected and inflamed, a condition called *otitis*, of which there are three main forms:

1) *Otitis externa* describes inflammation of the outer ear. This occurs most frequently in swimmers and is therefore also known as *swimmer's ear*.

2) *Otitis media* is inflammation occurring in the middle ear and

resulting from bacterial or viral infection. Treatment usually consists of antibiotics. Similar to this is *secretory otitis media*—also known as *glue ear*—a condition marked by the chronic accumulation of fluid in the middle ear and which is often treated by a relatively minor procedure during which a double-cuffed tube, called a *grommet*, is inserted in the ear drum to allow excess fluid to drain from the middle ear. Common symptoms of middle ear infection include moderate to severe pain and a high fever.

3) *Otitis interna*—also called *labyrinthitis*—refers to inflammation of the middle ear. Common symptoms include dizziness, an impaired sense of balance, and vomiting.

Naturally, any kind of ear infection needs prompt professional attention as without it the hearing may become permanently impaired.

Summing It Up

The process of hearing is a very intricate one and metamorphosing air vibrations created by sound into nervous impulses the brain can interpret involves several quite separate stages, all of which need to be functioning properly to provide normal hearing.

In the next chapter, we will be looking at both what is meant by "normal" hearing and how tinnitus interferes with this.

Chapter 3
Normal Hearing and Sound Perception

Before turning our attention to how tinnitus interferes with hearing, it's useful to begin by considering just what sounds someone with hearing that can be described as being "normal" should be able to recognize and differentiate.

The three main fundamental characteristics of any given sound and which determine what kind of sound it is are its pitch, loudness, and timbre, and the ability to clearly hear each of these constituent components varies greatly even in people considered to have normal hearing. Let us look at each of these components in turn:

Pitch

The pitch of a sound is how fast or slowly the object producing it vibrates—the faster the vibration, the higher the pitch of the sound will be. Generally, it can be said that the shorter or smaller the vibrating object is, the higher will be the pitch of the sounds it produces. For example, the strings producing the high notes found at the extreme right end of an acoustic piano's keyboard are much shorter than those producing the deep bass notes that are triggered by the keys at the extreme left of the keyboard. Equally, the notes available on a trumpet— which is comparatively small—will fall in a much higher range than those you can get from a tuba, a much larger instrument.

Naturally, in these days of synthesized sounds, the size of an electronic instrument no longer indicates whether it will be high- or low-pitched.

Pitch is measured by how many times the sound-producing source vibrates in a second, this measurement called cycles per second or *cps*, but also frequently expressed as "Hertz," a term often abbreviated to "Hz." One Hertz represents one cycle per second; 10,000 Hertz means that the vibrations repeat 10,000 times a second. A thousand Hz is also often shown as one kHz, this abbreviation standing for one kiloHertz with "kilo" denoting that the measurement is in units of a thousand.

Normally, humans can hear sounds occurring within the range of about 15 cycles per second to 20,000 cycles. However, it is common for the upper limit to become substantially reduced as you get older, the upper audibility mark falling perhaps to as little as half of that which you might have had when you were younger. By the way, the human ear can in fact usually detect sounds lower than 15 cycles per second, but what will be discerned will be an ill-defined rumble lacking any definite pitch and which may be felt or sensed rather than heard. Sounds above 20,000 cycles are, however, totally inaudible to the vast majority of adults although some rare individuals may be able to recognize them. Children can often hear sounds pitched as high as 40,000 cycles, but this ability begins to drop off by around 100 or so cycles a year once maturity has been reached.

Despite these limitations, the range of pitches audible to humans remains vast, covering in excess of 10 octaves. To put this in perspective, the range of a normal grand piano—one with 88 keys—is seven and a third octaves. Many animals, of course, can recognize much higher pitches and this is why the so-called "silent" dog whistle works: the sound it makes is pitched higher than humans can hear—hence it's silent as far as they are concerned—but it still remains within the range audible to a dog.

Just how the human detects pitch is not fully understood, but it is at least partly controlled by the cochlea, different parts of its basilar membrane appear to be stimulated by different pitches. There is little doubt, however, that the auditory pathway and the brain also play a major role in pitch recognition. So far, science has failed to come up with a totally credible explanation as to why some people have *perfect pitch*—that is the ability to pinpoint any note exactly—while others are relatively tone deaf and unable to distinguish with certainty between sounds that are pitched as much as an octave apart.

Various experiments have proved most people can improve their pitch recognition through aural or musical training, but this usually only results in an improvement in recognizing relative pitches—that is, whether one tone is higher or lower than another and how big the difference is between the two—rather than leading to eventual absolute pitch recognition, this remaining the dominion of those blessed with perfect pitch, an attribute usually present from birth although its presence may not be recognized until much later in life.

Incidentally, it's worth noting that even those who are said to be totally tone deaf are only rarely completely so, with most of them perfectly able to recognize great variations in pitch. Were it not so, then these people would have immense difficulties with the spoken word, which—even in English—relies at least partly upon rising or falling inflections to convey its full meaning, such as the pitch rising at the end of a sentence often indicating an unspoken but very real question mark. Pitch is even more important in many other languages, notably Chinese, where a word may acquire totally different meanings according to the pitch used.

Loudness

While the loudness of a sound is determined by the amount of energy it releases—banging a drum with great force will create a louder sound than tapping it lightly—just how that loudness will be perceived by the human ear will also be affected by the pitch of the sound. Not all pitches are equal as far as the human ear is concerned. It will hear some more clearly—and therefore more loudly—than others.

The ear's sensitivity varies greatly over its hearing range, and while there are also great variations from person to person, this is how it will operate in most people:

◆ The hearing will be most sensitive to sounds falling in what is called the "middle high tones range," this encompassing frequencies from about 1,000 to about 4,000 cycles per second. Man's ability to hear sounds in these frequencies is so developed that were it any greater we would begin to audibly discern the movement of air particles themselves.

◆ Hearing sensitivity drops off gradually below about 1,000 cycles. It is just as well that we cannot hear sounds below a certain pitch because otherwise we would be under constant attack from low frequency sounds produced within our own body, such as those resulting from bone and muscle movements.

◆ Hearing sensitivity also reduces sharply above the 4,000 cycles ceiling, and then does so much more rapidly than the drop-off in the lower bass. Incidentally, it is to deliberately counteract the ear's greater sensitivity to middle tones that hi-fis and many television sets have a "loudness control" you switch on when listening at low volume. What this control does is boost the relative volumes of sounds both in the lower bass and upper treble regions, so restoring the overall *perceived* balance more or less to that which you'd hear with the control switched off but with the main volume turned up higher.

To put the above ranges in perspective, the fundamental of the note middle C or *do* (located just to the left of the keyboard's centre) played on a correctly-tuned piano will vibrate at 256 cycles. As the number of vibrations doubles or halves an octave higher or lower, this means that a standard piano's highest note—the top C at the extreme right—vibrates somewhat more than 4,000 times a second and the instrument's lowest note—the A at the extreme left—vibrates 27.5 times a second, or nearly twice as fast as the average low pitch audibility threshold.

However, many sounds do not have a definite pitch like that produced by musical instruments and are instead a combination of many different pitches, these being so interwoven that no single specific pitch—or series of them—can be discerned. Sounds without specific pitch are known as *noises*, the word taking on a somewhat different meaning in this context, typical examples of which includes sounds like those made by boiling water or the clatter of horses' hooves.

Naturally, when the sound is a noise, the ear's sensitivity to pitch plays little role in determining how loudly it is heard.

The range of loudness to which a healthy ear can respond is vast, the ratio having been calculated as a hundred million to one, meaning that the loudest recognizable sound may be a hundred thousand thousand times louder than the faintest one which can still be heard.

Loudness is expressed in *decibels* (abbreviated as *dB*), a unit for indicating the relative intensity of sounds, which results from a logarithmic calculation applied to a measurement of the variation that a given sound source creates in the sound pressure of the air molecules. However, because the human ear has varying sensitivity to different ranges of pitches, the standard decibel measurement is usually converted to a different form that takes this into account, known as dB(A). It is this unit of measurement that is used most commonly to express loudness levels as they relate to human hearing. To put these in perspective, here are the approximate dB(A) levels for some common sounds, all of these based upon the assumption that the listener is comparatively near to their source:

 Only just audible ambient sounds, such as those you might hear on a still day if you really listened for them—10 dB(A).

 Whispered conversation—40 dB(A).

Conversation at normal loudness—60 dB(A).

 ◆ Shouting loudly—80 dB(A).

Symphony orchestra during a loud passage—100 dB(A).

 ◆ Jet airplane at full thrust, as during takeoff —in excess of 120 dB(A).

◆ Firing of medium-calibre rifle —160 dB(A).

Just where the thresholds of painful and/or harmful noise lie varies somewhat from person to person. Different experts also have conflicting views on this, but the following will serve as a point of reference:

It's generally agreed that damage to hearing may result following prolonged exposure to sounds in excess of 90 decibels.

Sounds in excess of 130 decibels are likely to be physically painful to endure as well as likely to cause damage.

It needs to be borne in mind, however, that the loudness of a sound is also related to the distance separating the listener from its source. In fact, scientists differentiate sharply between the intensity of a sound, this being a measurable physical quantity, and its loudness, this being the product of both the sound's intensity and how sensitive the ear is to it under the currently prevailing conditions.

Because our perception of loudness is also affected by our reaction to the kind of sound we're hearing, it can be difficult to state exactly at what level sound becomes obtrusive. For example, if you love Wagner's music you may well find the crescendo in the Ride of the Valkyries totally acceptable at 100 decibels. However, should the same relative level of loudness be produced by your neighbor's children playing the latest pop music, then you may well think of this as being excruciatingly painful.

Two other factors that affect just how "loudly" we hear something:

1) The human brain generally does an excellent job in filtering out what we want to hear from that which is of no or little interest to us—for example, a mother may well hear *her* child's voice more clearly than that of the other children when they're all singing at more or less the same volume in a choir; and

2) When there are many sounds of varying

volumes, the one with the consistently highest pitch will usually be heard most sharply even though its volume may be lower than that of many of the other sounds. This phenomenon explains why—apart from what the sound engineers may have done with relative volumes when mixing a recording—a singer's voice (which is usually mainly in the treble) soars distinctively above the accompaniment (most of which is in the bass and middle regions).

Timbre

The third major component by which a sound is identified, timbre is that quality which makes a particular sound what it is, or why a piano sounds like a piano and not a trumpet.

Virtually all sounds incorporate a number of what might be called sub-sounds, except that these additional sounds are in fact pitched higher than the one we hear most clearly. For example, if you strike the note middle C on a piano, the string struck by the hammer will vibrate at 256 cycles per second. However, apart from vibrating along its whole length, the string will also vibrate in halves—

the two halves, of course, being exactly half the length of the whole string will therefore vibrate exactly twice as fast, producing a fainter but still discernible note sounding exactly an octave higher than the one being played, this last being known as the fundamental. The creation of overtones doesn't stop at just halves because the piano's string also vibrates in thirds, quarters and so on, each of these subdivisions of the string producing sounds that are pitched higher and higher until they are so high that they can no longer be heard by the human ear.

The sounds produced by the vibrations of only a part of the string are called *overtones*, *harmonics* or *partials* and it is the relative volume of these that gives an instrument its peculiar and distinctive sound. For example, a good piano will produce quite strong overtones throughout the audible range, but a clarinet will produce almost no overtones. Of course, it is not only musical instruments that produce overtones as these are literally part and parcel of most sounds and one of the main reasons why we usually recognize them immediately for what they are. Because, by definition, overtones are pitched higher than their fundamental, it's quite common for some of these to fall in a range beyond that which we can hear, especially when our upper hearing range has become restricted. When that happens we may have difficulty in fully interpreting or understanding the source sound because we failed to capture enough of its overtones.

Another distinguishing mark of any sound is its *attack envelope*, a phrase that describes the manner in which the sound first manifests itself and then continues. Broadly speaking, there are two main types of attacks:

1) Percussive sounds are those which start off loudly and whose loudness then reduces rapidly. The piano and guitar are two common examples of instruments producing percussive sounds. Typical examples of nonmusical percussive sounds include thunderclaps or the snap of a twig being broken.

2) Constant sounds are those whose volume alters but little while they are being produced, such as those coming from a flute or a church organ.

There is also a third form of attack, one in which the sound starts off at low volume, then gradually becomes louder and louder. Incidentally, many sounds incorporate more than one form of attack, with some aspects of the sound gradually rising in volume while others remain constant or diminish.

Speech, of course, according to what is being said and how it is being said can be either mainly percussive or constant, depending upon whether the speaker adopts a staccato or sing-song delivery. The manner of speech, apart from whether the speaker has a high or low voice and speaks loudly or softly, will also influence the extent to which it may be heard clearly by someone whose hearing is less than perfect.

Sound Transmission

Of particular relevance to some forms of tinnitus is how sound can be transmitted. Generally, of course, the medium of transmission is the air, this responding to the vibrations created by the object making the sound, and the human ear is particularly suited to picking up airborne sounds.

Solids can, however, also act as excellent sound transmitters, one obvious example of this being the "listening sticks" used by water company inspectors to detect leaks in underground pipes. Similarly, the human ear may hear sounds which are brought to it via the bones or the tissues of the body.

Liquids, too, are good sound transmitters, as evidenced by how electronic devices can track down submarines many miles away. Equally, the liquids in the body, the main one being blood, of course, can act as a conduit bringing sound sensations to the ear.

Summing It Up

All sounds—and therefore all noises—consist of a number of different components, some of which may be more or less audible to a given individual, according to the state of his or her hearing. In the next chapter, we will be looking at the sounds associated with tinnitus, these generally having no obvious source.

Chapter 4
The Sounds of Tinnitus

In previous chapters we have seen how hearing works and what range of external sounds people with normal hearing would generally be able to hear.

While tinnitus is generally defined as "noises heard in the ear in the absence of matching noises in the surrounding environment," this definition is not complete because it fails to take into account that tinnitus can also be the result of hearing sounds that do exist, although not necessarily in the environment but rather in the body itself.

There are, of course, many forms of tinnitus—and experts have created a wide variety of labels to define its various subdivisions—but essentially the disorder can be broadly classified as to whether its manifestation matches one or more of the following four main categories:

1) So-called *objective tinnitus*—some forms of which are also known as *pulsatile tinnitus*—occurs when the noises that are heard are real enough, although

of a kind that most people do not hear. In these instances, the sounds can also be distinguished by observers and the source of the noises invariably lies within the body of the patient.

2) The phrase *subjective tinnitus* is generally used to describe a situation where the sounds heard by the patient, whether or not some of these may indeed still be the result of what might be objective tinnitus were their source only more amenable to independent observation, are such that they are not audible to someone else, no matter what equipment may be used to try to detect them.

3) Additionally, tinnitus whether objective or subjective, can be further classified upon how much it affects the patient. If the symptoms of the tinnitus are so negligible or happen so rarely that the patient is most often unaware of their occurrence and it causes him or her but little bother, then the condition is often described as *normal tinnitus*, a phrase that can also have a slightly different meaning as will be seen later.

4) On the other hand, the phrase *significant tinnitus* is, as you might expect from its first word, used to describe a situation in which the disorder is either frequent and/or noticeable enough to interfere to a greater or lesser extent with the sufferer's daily routine.

These general categories are not mutually exclusive. However, tinnitus will be *either* objective or subjective; normal *or* significant, the four possible main permutations within these categories are:

1) Objective *and* normal. In this case, the noises can be detected by others, but they have hardly any effect on the patient.

2) Objective *and* significant. Once again, the noises can be independently confirmed, but their effect upon the patient is great enough to cause discomfort, distress, or worse.

3) Subjective *and* normal. The noises are only heard by the patient, but their effect remains minimal.

4) Subjective *and* significant. Again, only the patient can hear the noises and they

have a considerable adverse effect on him or her.

Let us now look at the first two main types in greater detail.

Objective Tinnitus

The human body is a very busy place with all kinds of processes taking place all the time: the heart beats, the lungs expand and contract, foodstuffs make their way along the intestinal track, joints move, blood courses through the veins and arteries, and so on. Many of these processes are far from silent and the sounds they make can often be readily detected by an independent observer using a stethoscope or other sound-amplification device at or near their source. However, under most circumstances, the vast majority of people remain blissfully unaware of the noises made by their own body as it goes about its routine tasks, this happening for two separate but interconnected reasons:

1) The sources of many of the body's internal sounds lie in areas well insulated by surrounding muscles or other tissues, this insulation contains the vibrations created by the sounds and reduces their

intensity outside the immediate area of their origin.

2) Despite the muffling effect of any insulation that may be present, many inner body sounds can still have enough energy to fall within the audible range by the time they reach the ears. However, because the brain has a marvellous ability to discard or ignore information that's not considered relevant at the moment, many—if not all—of these sounds will simply be "filtered" out as though they didn't exist in the first place.

In fact, there is usually a third factor in play that also influences what body sounds are consciously perceived and which are not. As a generality, any such sound produced with regularity or more or less constantly will be ignored by the brain. It is, of course, very fortunate that this is the case because otherwise we would be conscious of hearing a thump with every heart beat or a whoosh of air whenever we breathed in or out.

Additionally, the brain's noise filtering mechanism also does an excellent job in recognizing when a normal body noise suddenly becomes changed for any reason. For example, someone with a slightly wheezy chest may be quite unaware of the sound this creates under normal circumstances, but should the wheeze change—although not necessarily become louder in absolute terms—the brain can stop its filtering of this particular sound, so making it audible and thereby drawing the patient's attention to it. In some ways, making a previous inaudible sound perceivable can be compared to the protective aspect of pain, both of these serving to draw attention to something which has gone wrong or which is no longer behaving normally.

There are many possible sound sources within the body that can lead to objective tinnitus, some of the main ones including:

◆ The circulation has frequently been identified as a source of objective tinnitus, and particularly likely to be heard is the flow of blood through the bigger vessels in the head or through the very small arteries that supply the ear, most specifically those leading to the inner ear. As already mentioned, the heart beat can be a source of tinnitus noise. This kind of tinnitus is usually comparatively easy to diagnose because the noise will almost invariably vary and decrease in loudness in close synchronization with the heart beat. Incidentally, it needs to be noted that being able to hear part of your circulatory system working is by no means an indication that there is anything wrong as such with the circulation. Despite that, it would nevertheless be sensible to have your doctor do a general checkup. In passing, it's worth noting that liquids such as blood are an excellent medium for the transmission of sound vibrations.

◆ Next to the circulation, the skeleton is probably the most common source of sounds that result in objective tinnitus. Whereas all joints can potentially produce noise, the most likely offenders include bones in the jaw, neck, back, and shoulders. Rarely will tinnitus stem from a distant joint, such as a knee, although this can happen. Usually, but by no means always, further investigation will discover that the "guilty" bones have suffered some deterioration, such as that resulting from arthritis. Some people, of course, just have bones that "click" more than the average, the sound produced being often loud enough to be heard quite clearly by anyone near them. Strangely enough, tinnitus seldom follows when the noise made by the bones is obviously audible.

◆ While muscles are a comparatively rare source of noises, those in the soft palate are an exception to this general rule, and tinnitus sounds have been clearly linked to their contraction.

Subjective Tinnitus

If no source can be identified for the noises heard by the patient, then the disorder will be described as subjective tinnitus. However, it is important to keep in mind that this is a label that may not truly reflect the facts. For example, just because no inner body origin has been found to explain the noises, this is far from absolute proof that there isn't such a source.

For example, some inner body sounds that have been shown as leading to objective tinnitus can be extremely difficult to locate, even with the help of today's extremely sensitive and sophisticated amplifying instruments. Obscure sounds like these would probably never have been identified a few decades ago when the equipment that can now track them down simply didn't exist, and the patient would have been diagnosed as having subjective tinnitus. It's therefore not unreasonable to speculate that there are possibly further inner body sounds that are so faint that their detection still remains beyond the power of modern gadgetry, but that these may eventually be identified by even more powerful equipment to be developed in years to come. Should this happen, then it's very possible that many a diagnosis will have to be revised, with cases previously labelled as being subjective tinnitus then falling clearly in objective tinnitus category.

Additionally, the phrase subjective tinnitus should never be interpreted as meaning the noises are *imagined* as almost certainly there is indeed a physical cause for them, even if that cause is not producing sound but instead leads to what can only be called the sensation of sound elsewhere. For example, as   explained more fully when we look at the causes of tinnitus, the disorder can often be linked to damage in some area of the body, this most commonly, of course, being one that is part of the hearing system. While the area that's damaged doesn't itself *make* a sound, it may nevertheless create nerve impulse that either the ear or the brain mistakenly recognizes as sound impulses. Just as those of objective tinnitus, the origins of the subjective variety can often be traced to specific physical malfunction or damage.

It's worth stressing the point made above because unfortunately the phrase "hearing noises in the head"—which is commonly used to describe tinnitus, even by people afflicted by the disorder—all too readily lends itself to misinterpretation that the noises aren't "real," that they're creations of the mind instead of being symptoms of something gone physically awry. The sensation of hearing sounds is real enough, even though the source of these sensations may itself not be a sound-producer, in that it doesn't create sound vibrations but instead sets off impulses or signals that are eventually perceived as sounds by the brain.

Significant or Not?

The dividing line between normal and significant tinnitus is one that gets very blurred at times because the extent to which someone may be affected by the disorder depends more upon his or her individual reaction to the noises than upon how loud they are or appear to be.

Statistical surveys of tinnitus sufferers have often shown there can be quite a discrepancy between how loud or constant a sufferer says the noises are and how much he or she is affected by them. It would be totally wrong to assume simply because a sufferer describes the noises he or she hears as faint or occasional that they are therefore of little significance. On the contrary, some of the people most distressed by tinnitus report the sounds they hear as being quite faint. Conversely, other patients who report relatively loud tinnitus noises say that they are not bothered greatly by them.

This lack of correlation between the loudness of tinnitus and how much it affects the patient occurs in both subjective and objective tinnitus. Incidentally, the very fact that loudness doesn't necessarily bring proportionate distress has provided a very important clue as to how tinnitus that cannot be cured can still be considerably alleviated, as will be explained fully in later chapters.

Naturally, how frequently the noises are heard has a great bearing upon their impact. As might be expected, if the tinnitus occurs but rarely, then it's usually much easier to bear than if it is constant or virtually so. However, interestingly enough, some sufferers from intermittent tinnitus have said that they thought it might bother them less if it were constant. One patient explained this view as follows: "It's bad enough when I hear the noises, but what is worse is not knowing when they may strike again.

When I'm free of the noises for a good while, I begin to hope that I've been cured. Then the sounds come back, and that is such a letdown that I wish they had never gone away at all if they weren't going to disappear forever."

Just when and for how long the sounds of tinnitus are heard by sufferers varies just as greatly as the nature of the sounds heard. At one extreme, some patients say their noises are with them all the time, even "hearing" them while they are asleep; others say the sounds only occur rarely, perhaps as infrequently as every few months. Most commonly, patients say the noises do abate now and then, sometimes for lengthy periods, with no obvious pattern to their presence or absence.

Finally, it should be noted whether tinnitus is significant or not in a given individual is not graven in stone. Tinnitus that began as "normal" quite commonly worsens into becoming "significant"; more rarely, the reverse may also happen, and when it does it's usually because the sufferer has learned to adapt to his tinnitus rather than the condition having improved to any great extent. Naturally, depending upon its cause, significant tinnitus can also respond dramatically to treatment, so reducing it to a level where it can no longer be called significant.

Incidentally, the phrase "normal tinnitus" is also used to describe that very temporary form of the disorder just about everyone now and then experiences in a comparatively minor way. People who do not have tinnitus as such are still quite likely to hear "noises in their head" for a little while after having been exposed to very loud sounds, such as having spent the evening in a disco. That kind of tinnitus, if that is what it really is, does however usually clear up of its own accord within minutes, or at worst within an hour or so, although there is some evidence to indicate that repeated experiences of this kind are likely to predispose to the development of true tinnitus later.

The Noises of Tinnitus

While almost any kind of sound may be experienced by a tinnitus sufferer, there are some that patients report time and time again, the more common of these including:

◆ Ringing sounds, ranging from those resembling a telephone's shrill ring to more sonorous bell-like noises. Ringing noises, of course, are classically associated with tinnitus, frequently described as "living with ringing in your ears" or the "ringing disease."

◆ Ill-defined sounds, somewhat like those made by a babbling brook.

◆ A hissing noise, usually quite high-pitched, resembling steam from the spout of a kettle coming to the boil.

◆ A buzzing noise, rather like that of swarming flying insects.

◆ Humming sounds in all their possible permutations, such as hums that sound like a muffled choir or like the background noise produced by a radio that's turned on but not tuned into a station.

◆ Clicking sounds of all kinds—including those like the tapping of the keys of an old-fashioned typewriter or the sounds made by a hot car engine as it cools down after having been switched off. The clicks may either follow a pattern, recurring at fairly intervals, or be totally random. Irregular clicking noises, of course, are often associated with objective tinnitus stemming from noises made by joints in the body.

◆ Whistling noises of all kinds—ranging from human whistling to mechanical whistles, with both the pitch and the volume usually remaining fairly constant.

◆ A throbbing noise, usually quite low in pitch.

◆ A noise that resembles a growl, except that it doesn't come to a natural end but continues indefinitely.

◆ Tweet-like sounds, almost birds' chirping.

Extensive though the above list is, it only covers a fraction of the noises that tinnitus sufferers have reported. In fact, it can be safely said that if you think of a sound, any sound, then it's almost certainly that someone somewhere experiences that sound as tinnitus. To further demonstrate just how varied tinnitus can be, here are some of the more unusual sounds reported as they were originally described by patients:

◆ Sometimes I think what I'm hearing is the noise of the earth turning on its axis.

◆ I keep hearing musical notes. All the notes have a very definite pitch and vary in length, just like those in a composition, but they never develop into anything even remotely like a tune.

◆ It's as though a group of very shrill-voiced children are shouting and yelling as they play their games in my head.

◆ I can't describe the sound I hear, other than it's very deep, very ominous, and almost threatening.

◆ It's just like being in the middle of what I imagine a railway shunting yard to be like: the clatter of heavy steel wheels on rails; the hissing and puffing of steam engines; and the clanking of freight wagons.

Although many people with tinnitus refer to noises that *sound* like those made by human voices, few indeed report these noises as voices, generally choosing to describe them instead as being "voice-like." Yet some patients do say they hear quite distinct voices that now and then speak words that are recognizable and which may or may not make some sort of sense.

Some experts have speculated that voices are heard by more tinnitus sufferers than has been revealed by various research projects, the reason for

this being that patients may be very reluctant to admit to hearing voices because this symptom is so
strongly associated with certain forms of mental illness. However, judging by what has been reported
by tinnitus sufferers who have said they heard
voices, the kind of words spoken by the inner voices
of tinnitus are very different from those heard by
mental patients: tinnitus patients generally appear
to hear random words, as though they were eaves-
dropping on a conversation, but only hearing part
of it; people with mental problems usually report
that the voices they hear are very clear, very definite, often speaking with great authority, as well as
issuing commands and demands.

Stereo or Mono?

Depending upon its causes, the noises of tinnitus
may be heard by the patient in both ears or only
one. In fact, as we'll see later, which of these applies
can be an important clue in determining what the
underlying cause may be. Occasionally, the noises
may shift from one ear to the other.

Much more rarely, a patient may report that he
"senses" the noises rather than "hears" them, the
sensation then usually appearing to be coming from
somewhere within the head.

Most commonly, tinnitus sufferers say that they hear only one kind of noise, although some of its characteristics may change at different times, become louder or softer, shriller or deeper, yet essentially remaining the same. Some patients, however, experience a whole gamut of different sounds, either separately or at times mixed together in total cacophony.

Summing It Up

Tinnitus can manifest itself in an incredible variety of ways, with the possible permutations of its symptoms being virtually infinite. Although, according to the symptoms it produces, the disorder can be classified into several main categories, a patient's individual experience of it is almost certainly unique.

In the next chapter, we will be looking more closely at the various causes of tinnitus and also at how the risk of developing it can be reduced.

Chapter 5
The Causes of Tinnitus and How to Prevent It

Before looking at the causes of tinnitus, it is useful to first of all consider exactly what is meant by the word "cause" in this context.

For example, it is known that tinnitus often follows prolonged exposure to very loud sounds, these eventually damaging parts of the hearing system. But which is the true cause of the resultant tinnitus? Is it the damage to the ears—or is it the exposure to the sounds that brought on the damage in the first place? There is no simple answer to that question and one could argue for forever as to which factor should be judged to be the cause of the tinnitus under those circumstances. Interesting though such an argument might be from an academic viewpoint, its outcome would not be of great help to someone seeking to reduce his or her risk of developing tinnitus, except for drawing the obvious conclusion that loud sounds are best avoided.

In this chapter, we will therefore use the word "cause" as it's generally understood by most people:

something which is seen as bringing about something else, the something else in this instance naturally being tinnitus. At the same time, we will be paying particular attention to those causes whose impact can be lessened by preventative measures.

In some cases it will be possible to clearly establish a cause for the tinnitus, such as when it's due to the taking of certain medications or because the ear canal has become blocked by compacted ear wax. In most instances, however, the immediate cause will be less obvious and may often be a matter of conjecture. One recent massive survey of nearly 1,000 tinnitus sufferers asked them what they *believed* might have caused or triggered off their tinnitus:

◆ Nearly a quarter of the respondents believed that their tinnitus was due to previous exposure to loud noises.

◆ Just under a quarter attributed their problems to stress.

◆ One out of every five sufferers said that their tinnitus was caused by having catarrh or being asthmatic.

Other causes frequently mentioned by patients include a history of hearing disorder (nearly 15 percent), accumulation of ear wax (six percent), and a operation not involving the ear (also 6 percent).

Causes that came up much more rarely included migraines and headaches, as well as having suffered a heavy blow on the head.

When the same patients were asked to list events that occurred more or less at the same time as the tinnitus first became noticeable, the answers suggested other possible triggering factors:

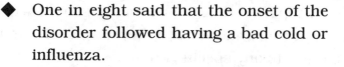 One in eight said that the onset of the disorder followed having a bad cold or influenza.

◆ Roughly ten percent said that loud noise had brought on the tinnitus; an equal number linked it to either Meniere's disease or vertigo. Somewhat fewer patients said that their tinnitus began when they became partially deaf.

◆ Other events mentioned frequently included an ear operation or ear infection (nearly nine percent), medical treatment with drugs or by injection for another problem (nearly nine percent), a blow to the ear or head (eight percent), preceding illness (nearly four percent). Interestingly, in this context, stress was only mentioned by somewhat less than four percent.

Events mentioned by relatively few sufferers included having their ears syringed to remove compacted wax or having had dental treatment that involved drilling (two percent), pregnancy (less than one percent, and the menopause (also less than one percent).

Additionally, just over 11 percent of the respondents reported that their tinnitus started without any warning whatever and they were unable to link its onset to any specific event.

Naturally, these statistics, based as they are on patients' personal views of their experiences, do not *prove* that the events reported actually caused the tinnitus, but they are certainly indicative. In many instances, of course, the cited events are those which can be proven to cause tinnitus, such as excessive noise or the accumulation of ear wax. Other events mentioned as causes are less susceptible to proof, such as stress or general illness.

The truth is that the cause of the disorder remains largely unknown in many cases of tinnitus. Yes, there may be some very strong pointers suggesting what brought it on, but absolute proof of the root cause will still often remain elusive.

Despite the above, there are, of course, many causes of tinnitus that can be clearly and unequivocally identified as such, and we will now look at the main ones:

Noise

The damage that noise can cause to hearing can be divided into two major categories:

1) Damage that is the result of a single incident involving a very high level of noise. Typical examples of this are explosions or gunfire. Usually, but not always, the hearing impairment will manifest itself relatively soon, if not immediately. Extremely loud noises can in fact totally destroy the organ of Corti in the inner ear, reducing it to fragments. Even death can be caused by a loud enough noise.

2) Damage that follows repeated and prolonged exposure to noise, such as working in a noisy environment or spending most evenings in a discotheque. This sort of damage usually takes a long time—years, even decades—before its effect becomes noticeable. Once again,

the organ of Corti is usually affected with some of the hairs cells having been destroyed, or the hairs themselves distorted, by the cumulative effect of noise exposure.

Naturally, it is not uncommon for hearing to have become adversely affected by *both* kinds of damage or for it to be less than obvious what kind of damage led to the impairment. For example, someone who served in the Armed Forces and at the time was exposed to the sound of gunfire may later work in an automobile assembly plant. Should his hearing start to fail some time thereafter, it would indeed be difficult to state with any certainty the extent to which either of these factors were to blame. One of the difficulties with linking cause and effect in many types of hearing problems is that the disorder is often insidious, worsening ever so slightly and gradually that it may take years before the patient becomes acutely aware that something is wrong.

Naturally, the way to prevent noise-induced hearing damage is to avoid noises loud enough to cause it, something that isn't always possible. However, these suggestions may help:

◆ Wear the right kind of ear protectors

when operating noisy machines.

◆ If your work environment is a noisy one, be sure that all governmental regulations about maximum noise levels are obeyed.

◆ When listening to personal radios or cassette players through earphones, always switch on the equipment and reduce the volume before placing the headset over your ears. Putting on the earphones first and then switching on may unleash a sudden blast of high-intensity sound.

◆ If rock concerts—or other equally loud entertainments—are your pleasure, avoid being too near the stage—the nearer you are, the greater the possible injury inflicted on your ears.

◆ If you are persistently and unavoidably exposed to loud noise—such as being a train driver—then make sure you have your hearing monitored at regular intervals. And should you ever experience the slightest ringing in your ears, then take this as a warning sign that it might be the first indication of tinnitus and immediately seek professional advice.

The Ageing Process

Even without the harmful effects of excessive noise, it is a sad fact that hearing normally deteriorates with the passing of the years. As was noted previously, what happens most commonly is that high-pitched sounds are no longer heard as clearly as before, if at all. Initially, this loss usually doesn't matter all that much for most people because the sounds they can no longer hear are usually not all that important to them. However, as the condition progresses and begins to affect the middle range— that region between about 500 and 3,000 Hz, where most speech falls—then there may be difficulty in recognizing words or parts of them. In spoken English most consonants are usually pitched higher than the vowels and therefore the first noticeable sign of hearing loss may well be an occasional inability to hear consonants. Another classical indication of hearing loss is difficulty in separating sounds, such as having trouble segregating one voice from the others in general conversation involving several people.

It can be difficult to differentiate between what might be called "normal" hearing loss, this due to the ageing process, and that which has been exacerbated for other reasons, but as a generality the following can be expected, this being subject to great variations from individual to individual:

◆ The symptoms of normal hearing loss seldom become apparent before the age of sixty years, although it will in fact be the result of a very slow process that have been at work for decades. This hearing loss, like that from many other causes, is invariably due to the degeneration of the hair cells and the nerve fibres in the organ of Corti, the damage being restricted to that area where the higher tones are perceived.

◆ Once the deterioration has become noticeable, it will appear to progress more rapidly and relatively few people older than seventy will still be able to distinguish sounds much higher than the highest note on a piano.

Loudness Recruitment

A curious effect known as "loudness recruitment" normally accompanies hearing impairment that's due to inner ear damage. Recruitment is characterized as:

◆ The hearing will be poor when the sounds are of low intensity, intensity of course also being related to the distance separating the listener from the source.

◆ The hearing will improve drastically as the intensity of the sounds increase, this improvement being much greater than that which would normally accompany the increase in intensity.

In other words, someone with loudness recruitment experiences larger variations in the volume of what he or she hears than those actually present in the sounds. Just why this phenomenon occurs is not fully understood, but some experts put it down as the brain increasing the ear's sensitivity across the currently audible range of frequencies to make up for the loss of those frequencies which are no longer heard clearly. Useful a stratagem though recruitment may appear to be at first glance, it in fact creates more problems than it solves because it overemphasizes the normal volume variations in ordinary speech and can make it more difficult for an affected person to hear it properly. Recruitment is one of the reasons why if you slightly raise your voice when speaking to someone whose hearing you know to be impaired, you may be accused of shouting at him or her.

Recruitment is also believed to be a frequent contributor to tinnitus, the increased sensitivity it creates in some frequencies leading to the hearing of sounds whose intensity would otherwise have been too low to have been noticed. Although recruitment is difficult to explain, it can be compared to what happens when you turn up the volume control on a stereo: as the overall volume from the speakers increases, it also becomes easier to distinguish any background hiss or static that may be present. Similarly, some forms of tinnitus are believed to be the result of the ear's "volume control" being turned up so high that previously ignored background noises are now discerned.

Ear Wax

Ear wax—its medical name is *cerumen*—normally plays a key role in protecting our hearing from damage, but as everyone knows too much of a good thing can quickly become a bad one, and ear wax is no exception to that rule.

Under normal circumstances, ear wax—which is produced by modified sweat glands in the skin lining our outer ear canals—fulfills several important purposes:

◆   It provides a barrier against possible infection, trapping dust and small foreign particles.

◆   It helps keep the ear canals supple while at the same time repelling excess moisture.

◆   It also acts as a "trap" for any insect invading the outer ear, the intruder gets stuck on the wax before it can reach the ear drum where it could do greater damage.

Despite ear wax's beneficial role, it can be a source of hearing problems when for one reason or another it accumulates or becomes compacted or hardened. Generally, the ears will clear themselves of wax, but occasionally this automatic process will fail to do a good enough job and the wax can then cause deafness and/or tinnitus. Fortunately, both conditions can be cured by removal of the wax, something that can be accomplished in several ways. However, before looking at these, a warning: **Never introduce any instrument whatsoever in your ears in an effort to clear wax.**

There are three good reasons for this admonition: firstly, probing about in the ear is almost certainly going to compress what wax there may be there, making it all the less likely that nature's own way will eventually clear it; secondly, whatever you use, be it a cottonbud stick or the wetted corner of a towel, is likely to irritate the ear canal's lining, making it secrete more wax than normal and so compound the problem; finally, there's a good possibility you may end up rupturing your ear drum!

Although there are various across-the-counter preparations you can buy to help shift recalcitrant wax, truly the best thing to do if you have a hearing problem you believe is caused by wax is to consult your doctor. That way you will not only almost certainly receive confirmation of your self-diagnosis but also have any other possibility eliminated. What's more, your doctor will arrange to have the wax removed safely by a nurse.

There are several methods for removing wax:

◆ Still most commonly used is an ear syringe, an instrument consisting of a cylindrical metal body with a spout at one end and a plunger at the other. The syringe is filled with warm water, the spout applied to the ear, and the nurse pushes the plunger, propelling the water into the ear where its pressure loosens and washes away the wax.

◆ A more modern version of the old-fashioned ear syringe is an instrument remarkably similar to the water picks used to massage gums or clear away food debris between the teeth. Like the dental pick, this syringe uses a jet of pulsating water, whose intensity can be controlled. One big advantage of this method is the pick is small enough so it can be observed while it does its work in the ear, therefore allowing the operator to direct it exactly where it's needed.

◆ Perhaps the best way of removing wax is the "dry method" in which a delicate probe is used to pry it away and break it up, the fragments then being sucked up by a miniature vacuum pump. Unfortunately, this method is not generally available at most local surgeries.

The following tips can help prevent wax from building up to the point where it becomes troublesome:

◆ Put a couple of drops of slightly warmed —not hot!—olive oil in each ear about once a month to stop the wax from forming a solid plug. The easiest way to do this is to stand in front of a mirror, tilt your head to the side, then use an eye dropper to let the oil fall into the ear. Place a little bit of cotton wool (make sure this is big enough not to be able to actually enter the ear canal but is just jammed at its opening) in the outer rim of the ear for about twenty minutes to stop the oil from coming out before it's done its work.

◆ Water entering the ear can swell any wax there and compact it. To avoid this happening: wear earplugs when swimming; plug your ears with cotton wool before showering or shampooing; make sure that your shower spray is never aimed directly at your ear opening.

While ear wax can be a direct cause of tinnitus, it has also been suggested that syringing compacted wax can set off the problem as many tinnitus sufferers have reported their problems began just after their ears were syringed. Despite the vast amount of anecdotal evidence to support this idea, medical experts do not believe syringing leads to tinnitus, offering two possible explanations why the two may appear to be linked as cause and effect:

◆ The patient's hearing was already susceptible to tinnitus before the wax build-up and the disorder would have developed in any case, its onset shortly after syringing being almost certainly purely coincidental; and/or

◆ Wax—especially if it has collected on the ear drum rather than merely blocking the ear canal elsewhere—can create tinnitus. Once someone experiences the disorder, he or she become more aware of its symptoms and because of this increased awareness may now hear faint tinnitus that previously went unnoticed although it may have existed long before there was a problem with ear wax.

Otosclerosis

This is a primarily hereditary disorder that often develops from late adolescence, then generally manifests itself in later life when extra bone formation occurs in the inner ear, this overgrowth leading to restricted movement of the ossicles in the middle ear, the stapes usually being most severely affected, even to the extent of becoming fixed to the oval window. Unless treated, the condition is progressive, leading to gradually deeper deafness as the transmission of sound vibrations becomes more and more impeded.

Tinnitus frequently accompanies developing otosclerosis although it is also possible for a patient to have the two conditions simultaneously, each being due to independent and separate causes. If tinnitus is present as a result of otosclerosis, then the noise it produces will usually be low-pitched.

Apart from tinnitus, another common symptom of otosclerosis includes hearing sounds as being "distorted," this distortion occurring long before loss of hearing becomes noticeable. The disorder is also frequently marked by patients reporting that their hearing is at its worst in quiet surroundings and appears more acute in noisy environments. Comparatively rarely, the condition may also be marked by vertigo.

Apart from using hearing aids to enhance the impaired sound recognition, otosclerosis can also be treated by *stapedectomy*, a surgical procedure replacing the stapes by a small plastic piston that performs the same job. Stapedectomies are usually very successful in restoring hearing, but they do not always also clear up any tinnitus present.

Meniere's Disease

Usually affecting only one ear and relatively uncommon in people under 50 years old, Meniere's disease—also known as *Meniere's syndrome*—is a disorder of the inner ear, its main symptoms include deafness, tinnitus, vertigo, and vomiting.

The symptoms are brought on by a substantial increase in the amount of fluid in the semicircular canals in the inner ear that help control balance and determine body position. The extra fluid damages the canals and, at times, also the cochlea, so interfering with sound perception and sometimes causing tinnitus. Unlike most other forms of deafness, the one that marks Meniere's normally primarily affects low frequency sounds, the loss usually being accompanied by loudness recruitment.

Most commonly, the first sign of the disorder is a sudden attack of vertigo, this at times being so severe that the patient may collapse. Attacks are occasionally preceded for a few days by discomfort or pain in the ear or tinnitus. How long attacks last and how often they occur varies greatly, but in most cases the deafness and tinnitus will persist between them.

The cause of Meniere's remains unknown in about half of the cases, the others being attributed to a variety of factors, including food allergy, congenital or acquired syphilis, viral infection, low activity of the pituitary, adrenal or thyroid glands, diabetes, and high blood pressure.

If a cause of the disorder can be identified, treatment will usually be addressed to rectifying the underlying problem. Other forms of treatment include drugs—notably *betahistine hydrochloride*, trade name *Serc*—which can lead to a reversal of the symptoms in the early stages of the disease. Left untreated, the condition invariably worsens, although the vertigo and the tinnitus may disappear as the deafness deepens or becomes total.

High Blood Pressure

There is a considerable amount of debate about the extent to which hypertension—that is having blood pressure that is higher than the normal for someone of the same age—contributes to tinnitus. Certainly, if the hypertension leads to Meniere's disease, then the link with tinnitus is proven. In many other instances, however, the connection is more tenuous, consisting mainly of the observation that many patients with tinnitus also have hypertension and that the former may improve when the latter is treated.

Whatever the effects of hypertension on tinnitus in general, there are aspects of it that clearly can influence tinnitus in two very specific ways:

1) Blood being pushed around the body at higher than normal pressure may create more intense sounds. If the tinnitus is of the pulsatile variety, that is its noises occur in synchronization with the pulse, then it seems likely that the louder the sounds made by the blood are, the more likely these will be heard as tinnitus.

2) The tinnitus may be the result of the blood being pushed that much harder through the very fine arteries that supply the ear itself.

If you have tinnitus for no other obvious reason and are also hypertensive, then it may well be that your hearing disorder will improve if you take steps to reduce your blood pressure. Equally, it seems logical—although not proven—that following a life-style that reduces the risk of hypertension may also reduce your chances of getting tinnitus.

Although it is beyond the scope of this book to go deeply into hypertension, here are some suggestions that can help either prevent it or reduce it if already present:

◆ Although severe hypertension may need drug treatment, milder instances can respond remarkably well and rapidly to making simple life-style adjustments, including keeping your weight down, getting more exercise, reducing your alcohol intake, and stopping smoking.

◆ Mental stress and anxiety are strongly linked to raised blood pressure and these can also be factors influencing how much tinnitus affects you. Simple programs to reduce stress and promote relaxation are described in detail later in this book and these can provide a dual benefit by helping you cope better with tinnitus as well as reduce your blood pressure if it's too high.

Apart from being a factor in tinnitus, hypertension also creates a substantially higher risk of eventually developing heart problems, having a stroke, and can also lead to many other serious diseases— all good reasons why it's a good idea to have your blood pressure checked regularly by your doctor.

Tinnitus as a Symptom of Another Disorder

Tinnitus is also associated with a number of other diseases or conditions. Not uncommonly, tinnitus is the "presenting symptom," the problem that brought the patient to seek medical help in the first instance. While a complete list of disorders including tinnitus as one of its symptoms is virtually endless, here are some brief notes about some of the main ones:

◆ **Tumors**—The word "tumor" merely indicates an abnormal swelling, usually due to an abnormal growth of tissues, in or on part of the body and does not by any means indicate cancer as a tumor may be benign or malignant.

There is one kind of benign—that is non-cancerous—tumor called an *acoustic neuroma* that creates tinnitus because it occurs in the fibrous sheet that covers the eighth cranial nerve, the one that links the inner ear with the brain. Tinnitus stemming from this cause is also usually accompanied by vertigo because a branch of the affected nerve also carries the signals from the organs of balance in the ear. Almost invariably only one ear is affected. While acoustic neuromas can be removed by surgery, this procedure only produces noticeable relief from any associated tinnitus in about half the cases.

◆ **Thyroid Problems**—The thyroid gland controls the body's metabolic rate by releasing various hormones. Both an over active or an under active thyroid—respectively *hyperthyroidism* or *hypothyroidism*—can be marked by tinnitus.

◆ **Diabetes**—Already mentioned as a possible cause of Meniere's disease, diabetes is a condition in which the body's cells fail to properly taken in glucose as fuel due to a shortage of insulin. Various researchers have pointed out that a much higher proportion than might have been statistically expected of tinnitus sufferers are also diabetics.

◆ **Multiple Sclerosis** (also known as *disseminated sclerosis*)—A chronic disease of the central nervous system, multiple sclerosis mainly affects young and middle-aged adults. MS, whose underlying cause remains unknown, causes damage in the myelin sheaths surrounding nerves in the brain and the spinal cord. If the disorder spreads to nerves linking the brain and the ears, then tinnitus may follow.

◆ **Meningitis**—Tinnitus may be the first symptom of meningitis, an inflammation of the meninges (the three connective tissue membranes that line the skull and vertebral canal) caused by viral or bacterial infection. Other common symptoms of meningitis include severe headache, rigidity of muscles, depleted appetite, and, in severe cases, convulsions. Treatment varies according to the cause with bacterial meningitis responding to antibiotics and sulfonamides while viral meningitis requires prolonged bed rest.

◆ **Head Injuries**—As might be expected, injuries to the head—especially if surgery was required to deal with them—are often linked to immediate or later onset of tinnitus. Because of the number of variables involved, it is often less than clear whether the tinnitus is a direct result of the injury or whether there already was a predisposition to the disorder.

◆ **Drugs**—Medications used to treat a variety of ailments can also produce tinnitus as a side-effect in susceptible people. For more information, see Chapter 7.

Summing It Up

Tinnitus can be due to a wide-ranging variety of causes and it can be difficult to identify which one may be responsible in a given case. In the next chapter, we will discover how tinnitus is diagnosed, its treatment then being matched to its cause.

Chapter 6
The Diagnosis of Tinnitus and Medical Treatments

Purists could argue that tinnitus is a symptom rather than a disorder or disease as such, and the noises associated with it are merely an indication that something is wrong, that something being the underlying disorder. However, in general usage the word "tinnitus" covers a much wider area than just that, denoting both symptom and disorder as required. The distinction can, however, be an important one because although one might say that someone is suffering from tinnitus, the fact may be that the patient has Meniere's disease and tinnitus is merely one of its symptoms.

While on the subject of definitions, it's good to clarify what "diagnosis" means in its strict definition when it describes the whole process involved in determining the nature of a disorder by taking into account many factors, the main ones include:

◆ **Symptoms**—these are problems the patient is aware of, such as being troubled by hearing noises which do not obviously match or are caused by sounds in the environment. It is the presence of one or more symptoms that normally leads a patient to seek medical help.

◆ **Signs**—these are indications pointing to a particular disorder which are recognized by the doctor but which are not apparent to or recognized by the patient. For example, someone complaining of hearing noises may not be aware there is an accumulation of wax in the ear, but the doctor will soon spot this as a sign of the underlying problem. Incidentally, this particular example illustrates that a given occurrence is not necessarily either a symptom or a sign. Had the hypothetical patient above noticed the wax himself and reported this to his doctor, then the presence of wax would have been a symptom instead of a sign.

◆ **Medical background**—naturally, what problems a patient may have had in the past can provide a vital clue to determining what it is exactly that's troubling him now, especially if the current difficulty appears to be a repetition of a previous similar episode. To continue with the example, if the patient with compacted wax complained of diminished hearing also revealed that his ears had to be syringed in the past, it would be pretty obvious where the origin of the problem was likely to be found. Of course, the clues that may be revealed by taking a patient's medical history are seldom that obvious and usually require a great deal more detective work to unravel.

◆ **The results of laboratory or other tests**—required tests are determined by the initial examination findings, during which a tentative diagnosis may already have been reached, the tests requested mainly for confirmation. In other instances, tests are required to exclude certain possible causes of symptoms, thereby reducing the number of conditions to consider. When tinnitus is the main or only symptom, tests of various kinds can play a major role in making a *differential diagnosis*—a diagnosis of a condition whose symptoms and/or signs also mark other conditions. As we saw earlier, tinnitus can be the first symptom of a number of disorders. It's obviously of vital importance to find out which is the underlying problem.

Naturally, not every case of tinnitus is investigated in such depth as in many instances it is very clear just what the matter is and what can be done about it. It is unfortunately only too true that not all tinnitus sufferers get all the help that's available, this at times being due to their own failure to press hard enough for expert attention.

To start at the beginning of the medical process, someone experiencing tinnitus will almost invariably first turn to his to her family doctor.

With tinnitus—as with so many other complaints—general practitioners have the unenviable task of acting as a clearing house, determining and judging whether a particular case lies within their own competence or if it needs to be attended to by a specialist. While there are no hard and fast guidelines to cover this, it would be most unusual for a GP not to refer a patient with ongoing and marked tinnitus—unless this were due to compacted ear wax or some other similarly obvious and curable cause—to the Ear, Nose and Throat (ENT) department of the local hospital. It also needs to be noted that some GPs do have to be coaxed somewhat before they will provide a referral, especially when the condition is mild. For those sufferers who might be reluctant to put pressure on their family doctor, it's well worth remembering that a hearing problem that remains less than fully diagnosed and therefore not treated as effectively as it might be can only be expected to become worse, a curable condition possibly becoming an incurable one with the passage of time. It is therefore sensible to insist on being referred to a specialist if your tinnitus fails to improve after treatment provided by your GP.

Preparing for a Consultation

Having been referred to an ENT specialist, the chances are you may well have to wait quite a while before your appointment. In the meantime, it is quite a good idea to keep a note of how your symptoms are progressing on a day to day basis as this information can sometimes help identify the cause of your troubles, such as for example whether the noises are triggered by specific events, these often but not invariably being sounds.

It can also be useful to jot down other things which may or may not be connected with your tinnitus, such as other health problems you experience, what medications you take, and also whether there are any periods of high stress or bouts of anxiety and/or depression. Of particular importance, of course, is anything which occurs shortly before or at the same time that your tinnitus is at its worst. Equally important can be anything that seems to alleviate the severity of the problem.

What Happens During a Consultation

Although individual consultants will have their own preferred approach, you can expect your initial examination to proceed more or less along set lines, beginning with an interview, then a physical examination and a brief check of some basic hearing functions, followed perhaps by some more questions after which you may be offered a diagnosis, this possibly only being a tentative one that will be subject to confirmation by further tests.

The Questions You're Likely to be Asked

After having taken some down some general details about you, the consultant will then ask specific questions relating to your problems, the areas covered at this time including:

Your general medical history, including possibly that of immediate members of your family as well.

 What medications you're taking currently and which ones you've taken previously. Medications include both prescribed medicines and those you've bought without a prescription.

 If any jobs you've ever held might have created a special risk of hearing damage.

Then questions dealing directly with the problem:

 How long have you experienced the difficulties?

 Are both ears affected? And if so, to the same extent? If only one ear is affected, which one? Is the tinnitus "sensed" elsewhere than in the ears? Is there or has there been discharge from the ears? If so, what form did it take?

 Are the hearing difficulties accompanied by pain or discomfort? All the time or only occasionally? How severe?

 Are the problems constant or only come up now and then?

◆ Does the severity of the condition vary greatly at various times?

◆ Did the problem come on all at once? Or was there a period over which it developed gradually, perhaps even almost imperceptibly?

◆ What is sound like? Is it high-pitched, low-pitched or just a vague noise without any apparent specific pitch?

◆ Have you ever experienced vertigo (dizziness)? If so, do you suffer all the time, frequently, or only occasionally? How severe is the dizziness? Does it merely make you feel somewhat unstable or does it lead to actual loss of balance?

Depending upon his tentative conclusions so far, the consultant may go on to a further list of questions, these possibly including:

◆ Have you noted any events which seem to make the problem worse or better?

◆ To what extent is the problem affecting you other than just physically? Does it make you anxious or depressed? If so, how severe is the anxiety or depression?

◆ Do you frequently have severe headaches or migraines? Any problems with your eyesight, such as double vision, blurring, loss of peripheral vision? Any difficulties in controlling your limbs? Any numbness or reduced sensation in any part of your body? Any difficulties with your speech? Do you have lapses of memory?

In most cases, the consultant will have a pretty good idea of what is the likely cause of the problem. But almost invariably, no opinion will be offered at this time. He will proceed directly to the next stage.

The Physical Examination

Depending upon the circumstances, this may be divided into three areas: an examination of aspects of your body that aren't obviously thought as being linked to hearing difficulties; an examination of the ears; and some simple tests to determine how well your hearing is working.

While tinnitus may be the specific reason why you've been referred to a consultant, the examination will nevertheless cover all aspects of your hearing. The reason for this is simple: tinnitus is frequently accompanied by deteriorating hearing or partial deafness, the impairment, however, being

often so slight or its onset so gradual that the patient hasn't noticed it. But, the existence or nonex-
istence of partial deafness will provide strong
evidence as to the likely cause of the tinnitus, many
forms of which can improve dramatically once any
underlying deafness has been treated.

If the consultant thinks that your hearing problem may be a symptom of some other disease, he
will look for signs that might confirm the presence
of another disorder. For example, should he think
your tinnitus stems from hypertension, he will
check your blood pressure.

In the absence of the likelihood of another underlying problem, the consultant will proceed directly to a visual examination of the ear, this
naturally being limited to the outer ear. Once again,
how he does this may vary, but generally this is
what will happen:

◆ The consultant will usually begin by
looking carefully at each auricle, the part
of the outer ear that lies outside the
head, pressing and probing gently, for
signs of inflammation, discharge, or undue tenderness.

◆ He will then inspect your ear canals, almost certainly using an *auriscope* (also

known as an *otoscope*), a hand held device that includes a funnel (the speculum) that is introduced into the ear, a battery-powered source of light, and an array of lenses to a clear view of the inside of the outer ear. Alternatively, the visual inspection may be carried out with the aid of a microscope. Either way, the consultant will be looking for evidence of excessive wax, inflammation or discharge, as well as anything indicating damage to the ear drum or ear canal.

◆ Finally, he will check whether your Eustachian tubes are opening and closing properly, by asking you to blow your nose while keeping your nostrils shut, an action that should cause the Eustachian tube leading from the pharynx to the middle ear to admit air from the outside, proof of this is the ear drum bulging slightly; and then asking you to swallow, this allows the escape of air from the middle ear and is marked by the disappearance of the bulging in the ear drum.

Once the visual examination is completed, the next thing will almost certainly be a series of simple hearing tests. Just what these may consist of can vary greatly, some consultants choosing to carry out a whole battery of tests themselves, while others limit themselves to the very basic ones, letting trained technicians carry out any further tests that may be required. Most commonly, at least the following test will be done at this time:

◆ A tuning fork—a device resembling an elongated fork but with only two tines and of much more solid construction and which emits a note when its handle is struck—will be sounded and placed near your ears and also on the mastoid bone, this being the lower part of temporal bone of the skull. As the fork is placed in different places, you will be asked several questions: do you hear the sound? Is it heard equally by both ears? Do you hear the sound better when the fork is near your ears or in contact with the mastoid bone? As the sound from the fork loses intensity, at what stage do you stop hearing it? From your answers, your consultant will be able to deduce several important facts about your hearing, including whether your problem falls into the *conductive* category, that is its source is in the ear canal, ear drum, or middle ear, or whether it's *sensorineural*, its cause lying in the inner ear or the nerves that carry the impulses from the cochlea to the brain.

After the Examination

Once he has completed his examination, your consultant is quite likely to have a few more questions to ask. Usually, these will be aimed at confirming his findings; occasionally, he may ask you to explain in greater detail some of the things you touched upon during the first stage of the consultation.

In most cases, you will then be offered a diagnosis, although that may be reserved until further tests have been completed.

Audiometry

Although any form of checking someone's hearing could be called *audiometry*, this word is usually reserved to for tests involving electrical apparatus.

Modern day audiometers test hearing in great and comprehensive detail. While checking someone's hearing with a tuning fork provides valuable information very rapidly, the results are pretty broad and will not exactly identify in what range the hearing may be failing and the severity of the failure. While finding that a patient has a measure of deafness is an important finding, the exact extent of the impairment needs to be determined before remedial action can be properly planned.

As you'll recall from a previous chapter, the range of frequencies used by human speech is a comparatively narrow band of those that someone with perfect hearing can perceive. Although it may be desirable to be able to hear as wide a range of frequencies as possible, the fact is that hearing will be generally considered as adequate for most purposes providing it is sufficiently sensitive to those frequencies covered by speech. There is also another very practical reason why this band of frequencies is the one most taken into account: most hearing aids are designed in such a way that they will only bring substantial improvement within that range. What this means is that while any loss of hearing in other frequencies may be indicative of the nature of the problem, the testing of hearing will generally concentrate on those frequencies lying between 250 and 8,000 Hz, with an even narrower range than that only being checked sometimes.

Hearing is tested with an audiometer, an instrument capable of synthesizing different tones at varying frequencies at various levels of intensity, the sound—usually a pure tone somewhat like a continuous tuneless whistle—being delivered to the patient through close-fitting earphones that exclude ambient noise, or possibly through loudspeakers.

Two different but interconnected aspects of the hearing are measured during testing—what frequencies can be heard and how loud the sound has to be at different frequencies before it becomes audible—the results are plotted on two graphs (one for each ear) called *audiograms*. At the left side of each audiogram there is an descending scale—ranging usually from 130 to -10 dB—where hearing sensitivity is recorded; at the bottom of the graph there is another scale, this one covering the frequency range from just below 125 to just over 8,000 Hz.

During testing, the technician uses an audiometer to send out tones of varying frequencies and volumes, the patient signals—usually by pressing a bell button, but possibly verbally—when he detects the incoming sound. Most commonly, the test will begin with tones in the upper middle range—say between about 500 and 4,000 Hz. Typically what happens is the following:

◆ First to be tested is sensitivity at, say, 500 Hz, a signal at that frequency is transmitted to the patient at various levels of loudness so the lowest level where the sound is heard can be identified. Depending upon the technician, this may be done in two different ways: either by gradually reducing the intensity until the sound is no longer heard; or by starting with a volume setting that is so low the sound will almost certainly be inaudible and then gradually raising the volume until it is heard. Alternatively, a combination of both methods may be used to pinpoint exactly the patient's threshold of audibility is for a particular pitch.

◆ The same testing will repeated for the other frequencies, and the whole series will then be repeated for the other ear.

What emerges from this test is a clear graphic indication of the hearing in each ear, represented on its respective audiogram as a line, its peaks showing where the hearing in a given frequency is good, and its troughs indicating where it is deficient.

Audiograms, of course, need expert interpretation, but as a generality, good or acceptable hearing—this being broadly defined as that which will probably not be improved to any great extent by a hearing aid—will be indicated by the following:

◆ Sounds in the frequencies ranging from 125 to 3,000 Hz should be heard when their loudness was 20 dB or less. Most commonly, however, these will have been perceived at 10 dB or even less.

◆ While sounds above 3,000 Hz generally need to be louder than the above before they are heard, there usually is a fairly steep drop-off in sensitivity in the higher pitches. The extent to which the drop-off in the higher frequencies will be considered as "normal" will be partly based upon the subject's age.

Some of other factors that will be taken into account when interpreting the audiograms:

◆ The age of the subject. Some loss of hearing—not necessarily limited only to the high frequencies—being part and parcel of the way the natural ageing process affects most of us.

◆ If some of the readings for the high middle frequencies fall into the 20 dB plus range, then how many of them do so? For example, merely to find that *one* ear provides less than fully adequate hearing at only *one* frequency is usually not all that significant and does not of it-self suggest that the patient would re-ceive great help from a hearing aid. If the same defect is markedly noted in a group of adjoining frequencies, then a hearing aid is more likely to help.

Incidentally, it needs to be pointed that audiograms use "0" as indicating the threshold of hearing, this threshold being based upon a standard obtained by studying the hearing of a large number of young people with totally healthy hearing. Despite that, the threshold mark remains an arbitrary one with many people whose hearing is perfectly fine for everyday purpose failing to hear *any* frequencies at such a low level, requiring the sound to often be at least 5 or 10 or even more decibels louder. There are some people whose hearing is so very sensitive that they can detect some frequencies at lower in-tensities than 0 dB, that being the reason why a standard audiogram starts at -10 dB so that these quite rare occurrences can be recorded without the line going off the chart.

Additional Tests

In most cases, a standard audiometer test is enough to provide all the necessary data to enable a diagnosis, but occasionally, a *bone conduction test* is also requested. This is essentially similar to the test described above, except the sounds generated by the audiometer are not transmitted to the subject's ears through earphones but instead are sent to the mastoid bone through a small device clamped against it. Within the device, sound vibrations created by a miniature loudspeaker connected to the audiometer are translated into mechanical vibrations, these being applied directly against the bone via a tiny piston. Bone is an excellent transmitter of vibrations and those produced by the piston will be received by the cochlea (both of them, in fact, but the one nearest to the piston will perceive the vibrations much more clearly than the other).

As this system of transmitting sound vibrations bypasses both the outer and middle ear, tests carried out this way will pinpoint exactly what sounds are heard by the cochleas and/or transmitted via the hearing nerves. Much valuable information about the source of the problem can be gained by comparing audiograms obtained in the usual manner with those resulting from bone conduction testing.

Additionally, there are many other kinds of tests which can be done if circumstances warrant, the main ones include investigations to determine, amongst other things: how easily and smoothly the ear drum and ossicles respond to vibrations; air pressure in the middle ears, this provides information about whether the Eustachian tubes are working properly; and how well the *stapedial reflex* is working, this is the automatic reflex that protects hearing against very loud sounds in excess of 80 dB by tensing a small muscle linked to the third ossicle, reducing the intensity of the sound conducted further along the line to the cochlea.

The Diagnosis

When all the tests have been completed, your consultant will be in a position to make his diagnosis. At that time, there will be two main possibilities:

1) The tinnitus appears to be due to or is a symptom of some other underlying problem which can be cured or helped by medical treatment, such as inflammation, otosclerosis, thyroid problems, or Meniere's disease. Naturally, in that case, the relevant medical treatment will be offered with the hope that as well as

clearing up the underlying disorder it will also cure or reduce the tinnitus. A medically treatable condition will, generally only be found in about five percent of the cases; or

2) As happens in about 95 percent of instances of tinnitus, the examination and tests will have failed to reveal any medically treatable cause for the disorder, other than, as is usually the case, the disorder is also accompanied by hearing that is failing somewhat.

Depending upon your point of view, the fact that medical investigation usually fails to find a medically treatable cause in about 19 out of every 20 cases of tinnitus can be seen as either good or bad news. To look first at the bright side, this means that most instances of tinnitus are not the result of another disease whose eventual consequences may be more dire. The bad news, of course, is that most cases of tinnitus are not going to be cured by medical treatment. This last sentence, however, must not be interpreted as meaning that medically untreatable tinnitus cannot be treated, even possibly "cured" to the extent that its effects are no longer noticeable, just that the help for the condition will not come in a form that can be provided by medication or surgery.

Drug Treatments for Tinnitus

Just what nonmedical help is available to ease tinnitus will be covered in depth in the next few chapters. Before going on to these, we will take a brief look at some medical treatments, excluding those for specific conditions covered in the previous chapter, which have varying degrees of success in making tinnitus more bearable. Seldom are drugs prescribed for tinnitus alone and many of those mentioned have been mainly used in trials, the results obtained not always fully confirmed by further studies. It's also worth noting that the "British National Formulary," a regularly updated joint publication of the British Medical Association and the Royal Pharmaceutical Society of Great Britain that lists all drugs in common use together with suggestions when and how they should be prescribed, doesn't even mention tinnitus as such in its index although the condition is referred to in connection with other disorders.

◆ Barbiturates, such as Amytal, are normally mainly used as sedatives, to counteract insomnia, and to reduce anxiety, but have also proven of value in relieving tinnitus. Despite various studies, it remains less than clear how the beneficial effects are obtained in tinnitus, these being possibly due to either a reduction in stress and anxiety or a lessened perception of tinnitus, or perhaps a combination of both of these factors. Whatever the true explanation, barbiturates do work for some tinnitus sufferers. However, there are many good reasons doctors are usually reluctant to prescribe these drugs. Firstly, patients can quickly become dependent on them; secondly, the beneficial effects may soon decrease as tolerance sets in, the combination of these two factors all too often leading to a situation where the drug does little to aid the problem for which it was prescribed in the first place but is still prescribed to postpone the problems that may accompany withdrawal. Additionally, the long term use of barbiturates can lead to severe side effects, including permanent damage to the liver.

◆ Several studies have been done on the effect of lignocaine, also known as lidocaine, upon tinnitus. Normally these drugs are used as local anesthetics or for regularizing erratic heart rhythms, but it was found that injections of lignocaine and related drugs could bring substantial relief from tinnitus, even clearing it completely in some patients. Unfortunately, the relief is short-lived, most commonly lasting but a few hours. What's more, the drugs can lead to serious side effects, including confusion and convulsions. Because of this, most experts have concluded these drugs were not a practical treatment method for tinnitus although further research continues, much concentrating on a form of lignocaine that can be taken orally.

◆ Tranquillizers—such as diazepam or lorazepam—are quite frequently prescribed for tinnitus sufferers, although it is not believed these drugs have any effect on the disorder itself, their value being confined to enabling the patient to cope better with the symptoms. Although exact figures are lacking, it is believed that a sizeable number of tinnitus sufferers are receiving regular prescriptions for tranquillizers. Various studies have reported conflicting evidence about the value of such treatment. For example, one research project found two thirds of tinnitus sufferers were helped by taking a minor tranquillizer while other studies concluded the benefits of such a regime were outweighed by the risks of side effects and possible dependence. It seems the extent tranquillizers can help is an individual matter, although currently available facts strongly suggest these drugs are most likely to be of substantial benefit when a) the tinnitus is quite severe, and b) the patient also has other problems related to stress and/or anxiety.

◆ Tricyclic and related antidepressants are known to often exacerbate tinnitus, but paradoxically may help some sufferers. Once again, it is less than clear just how the drugs provide benefits in tinnitus, but some experts believe that this may be due to an anticonvulsive effect; others, considering the links between stress, anxiety and depression, find a simpler explanation. One intriguing aspect of these antidepressants is that they can help reduce oral and facial pain, this leading some researchers to speculate about just how they may also affect the nerves involved in the hearing process.

Summing It Up

The above are, of course, just a few of the drugs that have been tried in tinnitus. Unfortunately, none has to date proven itself sufficiently effective to be described as a treatment of choice. However, this does not mean that drug therapy may not provide valuable relief for many tinnitus sufferers, just that the results are often unpredictable and that any benefits have to be carefully weighed against the risks of side effects and dependence that any long-term drug regime usually involves.

In the next chapter, we will look at other ways of reducing the impact of tinnitus, especially by avoiding or reducing our exposure to things that may either trigger it or make it worse.

Chapter 7
Reducing the Impact of Tinnitus

While medical treatments are unfortunately only likely to be of great help for a relatively small minority of sufferers from tinnitus, there are many other ways in which the impact of the symptoms can be substantially reduced, even possibly completely eliminated.

These nonmedical forms of help fall into three main categories:

1) The identification—and thereafter the avoidance—of those things that may set off symptoms and/or make them worse.

2) Electronic devices, such as hearing aids and tinnitus maskers, that reduce the effect of tinnitus either by improving the hearing as a whole or minimize tinnitus by introducing other sounds that have a tendency to "cancel" them out. For more details, see the next chapter.

3) Different ways of seeking to alter how strongly the sufferer reacts to tinnitus, this hopefully leading to a lessened perception of the noises and thereby making the disorder more acceptable and less intrusive or disabling. These approaches, which usually rely heavily on methods to reduce stress and anxiety, are, in fact, closely interwoven with preventing the symptoms from arising in the first place. See Chapters 9 and 10.

In this chapter, we will concentrate on those things that for many people make tinnitus worse, if not necessarily cause it. However, before we proceed, a note of explanation and caution is in order:

Subjective tinnitus invariably manifests itself in a very individual way with probably no two sufferers experiencing it identically. Equally individualistic are the things that can make the disorder better or worse for a given sufferer. This means that the suggestions and recommendations that follow, although suitable for the vast majority of people with tinnitus, will not work in every case. For example, while giving up smoking will be probably help most sufferers, there are those for whom the stress of nicotine withdrawal may perhaps precipitate worse symptoms than ever before. Readers are therefore urged to consider the following facts in the light of their own individual circumstances.

Food Allergy and Tinnitus

There is little doubt that many instances of tinnitus are worsened by eating certain foods, whether this be due to a side effect of an allergic reaction to the food or a substance in the food causing a direct effect. Like tinnitus, food allergy is usually a very individualistic problem and there are no hard and fast rules that say that this or that food will make tinnitus worse for everyone.

Nevertheless, there are some foods that time and time again have been identified by tinnitus sufferers as worsening their symptoms and it would certainly be worth trying to avoid these for some time to see whether that makes any appreciable difference in your case. Incidentally, also mentioned are foods linked to hearing loss in general, as tinnitus and hearing loss often occur together, and improving hearing often reduces accompanying tinnitus. Foods most likely to be "offenders" include:

 Coffee, tea, and other drinks—such as colas—that contain caffeine, a powerful stimulant. Although caffeine's initial effect is that of a pick-me-up, this temporary boost is soon followed by a letdown, and researchers have found this see-sawing between mild highs and lows can heighten anxiety as well as bring on depression in susceptible people. Decaffeinated coffee and tea appear to have no effect on tinnitus.

◆ A similar effect to caffeine has been attributed to cocoa, which is mainly found in chocolate, pastries, cakes, and chocolate drinks, but is also often one of the ingredients of processed or packaged foods.

◆ Food high in saturated fats have also been implicated, these, of course, being likely to raise your cholesterol level, so possibly leading to hypertension, a condition strongly associated with tinnitus. Additionally, several studies have confirmed a link between sensorineural hearing loss and high levels of blood fats, this probably being due to high blood fat levels causing hearing loss by restricting the supply of oxygen and nutrients to the inner ear. Further research has shown that following a diet that's low in saturated fats provides some protection against hearing loss and can even help bring improvement for those who have already lost some hearing.

◆ Alcohol. The evidence about the adverse effect of alcohol in tinnitus is rather mixed: generally, studies have found that for most sufferers, drinking alcoholic beverages tends to make the condition worse, but some patients have reported that alcohol improved matters for them, albeit only temporarily. It's worth noting that alcohol, seen by many people as a stimulant, is in fact a sedative and that could explain why it may be beneficial in small amounts for patients whose tinnitus is strongly linked to anxiety or stress. Naturally, should you find that the odd drink now and then helps you, then there would be little point in giving up alcohol, unless there were other good reasons for doing so. Do, however, keep your consumption to a safe level, this having been defined as up to 21 standard drinks a week for men

and 14 for women, a standard drink being a half pint of beer, a pub measure of
spirits, or a glass of wine.

◆ Cutting your salt intake may reduce your
tinnitus, according to many sufferers.
Apart from being more spare with the
saltshaker, remember that many processed foods also have a high salt con-
tent and seek to avoid these.

◆ A high intake of sugar, say researchers,
can be instrumental in bringing about
hearing loss. Scientists believe this happens because sugar stimulates the re-
lease of adrenaline which can reduce the
oxygenated blood supply to the inner ear
by constricting the very small arteries
that supply it. Improvements in hearing,
as well as occasionally reduced tinnitus,
have been reported by some after reducing intake of sugar and other refined car-
bohydrates.

◆ Food allergy in general has been strongly
linked to frequent bouts of middle ear
inflammation, a disorder which, if left
untreated, can eventually cause damage
to the ossicles. In one major study in-

volving more than a hundred subjects with frequent or chronic ear infections, it was found that more than three quarters of them were allergic to one or more common foods. When the implicated foods were withdrawn from their diets, three out of four of the subjects had either no further ear infections or only experienced them very occasionally. The most common foods creating an allergic reaction were wheat and soya bean products, milk, eggs and peanuts.

The specific foods mentioned above are those which have often been implicated in tinnitus. However, judging from patients' own accounts, just about any food may be a source of trouble, there often being no logical explanation as to why eating a given food should exacerbate tinnitus.

If you suspect some of the foods you eat are making your symptoms worse, begin by eliminating a few of the ones listed above for a week or two. If that makes no difference, then eliminate another lot for a while, continuing in this manner until at one time or another you've temporarily eliminated all of these. Should none of this help, then you can try keeping a diary in which you note both the foods you eat and record the severity of your tinnitus. Do this for a couple of weeks and then look at your entries, analyzing and comparing them. If you're lucky, you may almost immediately spot a direct correlation between having eaten a certain food, say eggs, and experiencing worsening symptoms.

However, the link is often not as obvious as the one suggested above and you need to bear in mind that there could be a substantial period of time separating a food "cause" and its resultant event. As this time-lag can be as long as three days or even longer, it may require a lot of patient detective work on your part before a pattern reveals itself.

Some Foods that May Help

Several nutritional deficiencies have been associated with some kinds of sensorineural hearing loss and, by extension, with the development of tinnitus. While there is no absolute scientific proof that ensuring your diet contains an adequate amount of these nutrients will help with either hearing loss and/or tinnitus, this is obviously a sensible thing to do. Remember, however, that if you seek to make up a shortfall of any nutrient by taking supplements, you should first of all consult your doctor.

Associated with hearing loss are deficiencies of:

◆ **Vitamin A (Retinol).** Good natural sources of this vitamin include fresh vegetables (especially green or yellow), cod liver oil, liver, milk and butter.

◆ **Vitamin D (Cholecalciferol).** Good natural sources of this vitamin include cod liver oil, egg yolk, margarine and cream. Vitamin D is also produced by synthesis within the skin when this is exposed to sunlight.

◆ **Iron.** Good natural sources of iron include meat, oyster, liver, chicken and turkey. Note, however, that too much iron can be just as harmful as too little because an overabundance of it can increase the risk of arterial disease and heart attacks.

◆ **Zinc.** Good natural sources of zinc include lamb, pork, oysters, herrings, pumpkin seeds, eggs, milk, beans, yeast and brewer's yeast.

Drugs that May Worsen Matters

Both prescribed drugs as well as those contained in preparations available without a prescription can contribute to creating deafness and/or tinnitus, whether temporarily or permanently.

Additionally, many drugs that by themselves would do no harm can interact with other drugs taken at the same time for other conditions to create a new set of potential side effects—this possibility is, of course, one more good reason why you should always keep your doctor fully informed about any non-prescribed medication you've obtained yourself.

During one recent international symposium on tinnitus, experts listed more than a hundred drugs whose use had been implicated in either creating or worsening tinnitus, about half of that number having also been found to lead to hearing loss on occasions. It, however, needs to be emphasized that most of these drugs only affected the hearing of a very small minority of patients who took them, and that problems with many of these medications only arose when they were taken in much higher dosages than normal. What's more, how someone reacts to a given drug is often a highly individualistic matter, just as food allergy can be, and a side effect that may affect one patient very badly may leave hundreds of others taking the same medication completely unaffected.

Commonly used drugs that have been identified as causing and/or contributing to tinnitus include:

◆ **Aspirin.** This most common of all painkillers is notorious for its ability to create tinnitus, usually of the high-pitched variety, in susceptible subjects, but for this to happen the dosage usually has to be quite high, perhaps several times that recommended for ordinary usage, and the medication taken for some time. While it is not believed that the occasional use of aspirin at a moderate dosage will heighten the risk of tinnitus, it is obviously sensible to avoid this particular analgesic if you have hearing problems. Having said that, it also needs to be pointed out that some patients with well established and quite severe tinnitus have reported that taking aspirin has *helped* reduce their symptoms.

◆ **Ibuprofen and indomethacin.** There is some evidence, sparse but accumulating, that these drugs, commonly used to control mild to moderate pain and inflammation in rheumatic disease and other musculoskeletal disorders, may lead to tinnitus or worsen this when already present.

◆ **Antibiotics.** These are medicines that destroy or inhibit the growth of microorganisms and are commonly used to treat a wide range of conditions arising from bacterial of fungal infection. Although these drugs have literally proven to be lifesavers on countless occasions, they have been implicated in tinnitus, although there is no accepted scientific explanation as to why this happens. Nevertheless, the accumulated anecdotal evidence from tinnitus sufferers is so great there is little doubt that antibiotics can trigger tinnitus or make it worse.

◆ **Antidepressants.** The role of antidepressants in tinnitus is a curious one. First of all, as has already been indicated, they can be a vital part of the treatment for tinnitus when this is due to or worsened by anxiety, stress, and depression. In fact, there are now many experts who believe antidepressants are a better overall therapy for some forms of anxiety, including those specifically linked to tinnitus, than tranquillizers. On the other hand, there is plenty of evidence to show that antidepressants can create tinnitus, the condition usually but not always disappearing when the drugs are discontinued. The only way to find out whether antidepressants will help is by trying them if your doctor suggests you should. Naturally, tell your doctor immediately if your symptoms worsen. By the way, should you be on a prescribed course of antidepressants, do not discontinue these without your doctor's prior approval as serious side effects can occur during uncontrolled withdrawal.

◆ **Diuretics.** Also linked to producing or exacerbating tinnitus are diuretics, drugs that increase the volume of urine produced by promoting the excretion of salts and water from the kidneys. The more potent diuretics are used to reduce salt and water retention in heart, kidney, lungs and liver disorders; milder preparations are prescribed to treat high blood pressure as well as reduce intraocular pressure in glaucoma.

◆ **Quinine.** Only rarely used nowadays, quinine was once commonly prescribed to treat and prevent malaria, an infectious disease caused by the presence of a parasitic protozoa in the red blood cells. One of the drug's well-established side effects is *cinchonism*, a poisoning caused by too high a dosage of quinine (or similar alkaloids) and whose symptoms include ringing noises in the ear, as well as dizziness and poor balance.

◆ **Cannabis**. Although not a medicine in this country, it's seen as having no therapeutic value, but certainly a drug, cannabis—also known as marijuana or hashish—is prepared from the Indian hemp plant. Because its use is illegal and therefore largely unrecorded, the evidence linking cannabis to tinnitus is mainly circumstantial. There is no doubt that tinnitus-like experiences can be part of cannabis' hallucinatory and euphoric effects, but there is less certainty about whether such tinnitus may eventually become permanent.

Smoking

Experts agree that smoking is likely to worsen existing tinnitus, but there is greater scepticism about whether the habit makes any sizeable contribution to increasing the risk of developing the condition.

Several studies have shown that smokers with moderate to severe subjective tinnitus have often reported an improvement in their symptoms after they had stopped smoking for some time. There is, however, another side to that coin in that some smokers who tried to give up found that the stress caused by this made their tinnitus worse. It is, of course, open to speculation whether their symptoms might have improved had they persevered long enough with their attempt to reach the point where the long-term benefits began to outweigh temporary side effects.

Naturally, deciding whether or not to quit smoking is a very personal matter, but if you do try and succeed there is every chance that this will improve your tinnitus, as well as bringing the additional bonus of greatly reducing your risk of developing many serious diseases. Incidentally, it needs to be added that nonsmoking tinnitus sufferers have often reported their condition is worsened when they are exposed to other people's smoke.

Reducing the Harmful Impact of Loud Noises

Various ways to protect your hearing by avoiding loud noises were already mentioned in Chapter 5, but these recommendations dealt mainly with noises whose loudness was to some degree under your control. Unfortunately, in today's overcrowded towns and cities, many of us are subjected to noises from seemingly uncontrollable sources. As existing tinnitus is often aggravated by certain noises in the environment, here is a brief summary of what steps you can take to reduce noises that you consider to be a nuisance, bearing in mind that a *reasonable* level of surrounding noise is part and parcel of modern living:

1) If, as is so often the case, your neighbors are the source of the noise/s—such as playing loud music at all hours of the day—then the first thing to do is to approach them politely, explain the problem, and hope that things quiet down thereafter. Should this approach fail to bring results, your next step is to. . .

2) Contact the Environmental Health Department at your local authority who can

take action on your behalf if they believe the noise amounts to a statutory nuisance. Your complaint will generally be investigated by an Environmental Health Officer (EHO) who will normally seek to sort out the matter informally with whoever is creating the nuisance. Should this fail, the local authority can serve a notice on the originator of the noise—or the owner of the premises where it occurs—requiring abatement of the nuisance. If this demand is ignored, proceedings can be taken in the local magistrate's court (in Scotland, the Sheriff Court) where offenders can be fined up to £2,000 upon conviction, with further fines for every day the offence continues thereafter. Even heftier fines can be imposed in England and Wales if the noise emanates from industrial, trade or business premises.

3) Should your local authority choose not to institute proceedings, you can complain directly to magistrates in England and Wales, or, in Scotland, make a summary application to the Sheriff. These

procedures, although meant to provide a simple remedy, can nevertheless quickly become complicated and you may find that it will be useful to employ a solicitor to represent you.

4) An alternative approach, although also fraught with possible legal pitfalls, is to take civil action against the noise maker. Civil actions can become very expensive and you should certainly seek legal advice before embarking on this course.

Ideally, you should try to avoid recourse to the courts, your chance of success is greater if your local authority is prepared to act on your behalf. For more information, see the booklet *Bothered by noise? What you can do about it*, published by the Department of the Environment, and obtainable from your local authority, and *Neighbor noise problems—What you can do*, a very informative four-page leaflet obtainable from the National Society for Clean Air and Environmental Protection, 136 North Street, Brighton BN1 1RG.

Summing It Up

Most of the information in this chapter has been aimed at showing how you can reduce the severity of your tinnitus symptoms by following some simple recommendations. For many sufferers, the relief that can be obtained from these self-help suggestions may be enough to make their condition considerably more acceptable. However, there are also other ways of reducing the impact of tinnitus, including "masking" its noises with other sounds, as we'll discover in the next chapter.

Chapter 8
Hearing Aids and Tinnitus Maskers

As we have seen, deficient hearing and tinnitus often go hand in hand and one logical step towards possibly alleviating tinnitus is to improve the hearing by using an electronic aid.

While not all people with tinnitus also have hearing loss that can be helped by a hearing aid many of them do. In those cases, artificially restoring hearing through an electronic aid may also go a long way toward clearing up the tinnitus or making it less noticeable. Additionally, while tinnitus maskers—more about these later—are available as stand-alone devices, they can also be incorporated in many hearing aids, and should a hearing aid be indicated then there's a lot to be said for having a device that can provide both amplification and masking.

We'll first of all look at just what hearing aids are and when they are likely to be useful.

How Hearing Aids Work

Put at its simplest a hearing aid consists of three main parts:

1) A microphone which captures sound, translating its air vibrations into variations in electrical current; and

2) An amplifying stage where these variations in electrical current are magnified many times—the degree of amplification being selected by the user through a volume control—to produce an output signal that is considerably greater than the original input received from the microphone; and

3) An earphone—this being essentially a miniature loudspeaker—where the amplified electrical variations are once again turned into air vibrations, these being directed via the external ear canal at the ear drum.

Additionally, of course, there is a small battery that powers the whole system. Although all hearing aids operate on similar broad principles, there are vast variations in their capabilities and also in the way they are presented—small aids are often worn in the ear or just behind it, and larger ones, which are usually more powerful, have the microphone and amplifier contained in a separate box that's worn on the body with a thin cable leading to the earphone. Alternatively, miniaturized hearing aids can be fitted within the frames of spectacles.

But, no matter what their configuration may be, hearing aids all work on the same principle: they amplify ambient sounds, making them loud enough to be picked up by the deficient hearing. Useful though these aids can be, they do, however, have their limitations and therefore will not always work as well as might be hoped with some kinds of hearing impairment. Here are some of the main factors that will affect just how effective a hearing aid might be:

◆ Hearing aids are most likely to be of considerable help when the hearing loss lies mainly in the frequencies between 100 and 4,000 Hz as the instruments generally produce little or no amplification outside that band. This range is, however, not as restricted as it appears at first glance because it covers the frequencies used by normal speech, this usually being the sounds people with impaired hearing most want to be enabled to hear more clearly. Additionally, modern hearing aids also allow for the selective amplification of specific frequencies within that range, so providing a greater increase of volume to those frequencies where the hearing loss is greatest.

◆ While modern day electronics can create extreme amplifications, too high an output volume from a hearing aid can in fact cause further damage to what hearing is left. For most people, the problem won't arise as a moderate degree of amplification will be sufficient. Generally, hearing aids are most likely to provide maximum benefit when the loss is such that a gain of up to around 40 decibels is adequate. Should much greater amplification be needed, then there's a danger that this in itself may eventually lead to further hearing loss.

◆ The greater the amplification needed, the greater the likelihood the aid itself will become a source of noise. There are two ways this can happen: first of all, all amplifiers produce a certain amount of background noise. Usually this noise is so faint it isn't noticed, but as you turn up the volume so the noise is also increased. What's more the signal-to-noise ratio may worsen appreciably at high gain levels—"signal" denoting the sounds you want to hear. Secondly, the louder the output through the earphone, the more likely that some of this may also be picked up by the microphone, resulting in the phenomenon known as feedback. Feedback means the sound being output is also being fed back to the input, creating an endless loop of distorted sounds that get louder and louder.

There are two main sources of hearing aids: a) through the National Health Service, or b) from independent commercial suppliers. While NHS aids were once considered as bulky and unsightly, the newer ones do compare very favorably with those you have to pay for, there often being little, if any, difference in the amount of hearing improvement they can bring. To obtain an NHS hearing aid, you will have to be referred to an ENT consultant or a hearing clinic at your local hospital, who will then decide whether an aid is indicated in your case.

Alternatively, you may decide to buy an aid privately. In that case, here are a few points to keep in mind:

◆ Make sure that the supplier is reputable and that the dispenser is authorized to dispense hearing aids by the Hearing Aid Council, a statutory body charged with regulating the private prescription and fitting of hearing aids.

◆ Even when properly prescribed and fitted, hearing aids don't always work out as well as might be expected. It is wise therefore to try one out before committing yourself to buy. Most companies will allow a trial period, this unfortunately not always being long enough to truly assess an aid's merits as it can take several weeks or even longer before you get fully used to it.

◆ While most people are perfectly satisfied with their hearing aids, things can and do at times go wrong. Should you feel dissatisfied for any reason, the first thing to do is to contact your supplier as soon as possible. Should this approach not bring acceptable redress, the following may be able to help:

The Society of Hearing Aid Audiologists
    Plas Newydd Usk,
    Gwent NP5 1RZ

The Hearing Aid Industry Association
    16a The Broadway
    London SW19 1RF

The Hearing Aid Council
    First Floor, Ashton House
    471 Silbury Boulevard
    Central Milton Keynes,
    Buckinghamshire MK9 2LP

Hearing Aids and Tinnitus

Just how much relief from tinnitus may be provided by a hearing aid varies greatly, but it is expected that some improvement may follow for perhaps up to a quarter or even more of patients whose tinnitus had been accompanied by marked hearing loss.

It's worth pointing out any improvement in tinnitus won't always be immediately noticeable. As has already been pointed out, it takes some time to get used to a hearing aid and to learn how to use it for best effect, any tinnitus-reducing benefit perhaps only appearing once you're totally familiar with the hearing aid.

Tinnitus Maskers

The basic principle of tinnitus masking is a simple one: if you're bothered by a sound but can't eliminate it, then the presence of another sound may counteract or "camouflage" the first one so that it troubles you less, if at all.

All of us mask sounds—if we didn't, our lives would be quite intolerable as our brains would be assailed constantly by a barrage of all kinds of noises, most of which would be of no importance to us but which nevertheless would have to be recorded and analyzed. Were some kind of automatic filtering not applied by the brain to incoming sound data, the sheer magnitude of this information would soon lead to a sensory overload. However, the brain's ability to discriminate between important sounds and those which aren't allows us to concentrate upon those that matter while more or less ignoring the rest.

Much of this filtering activity operates automatically, probably as the result of countless generations of evolutionary change, but the brain can also quite rapidly adapt this process to meet specific circumstances. For example, someone living near a railway line may after a while become blissfully unaware of trains roaring by—the brain learns to pay little or no attention to these sounds, recognizing them as being unimportant at the time. While a railway line may be an extreme example of an "ignored" sound, we all both consciously and unconsciously ignore many sounds, such as those made by ventilation and heating systems, traffic noises, noises made by co-workers in an office and so on.

The brain's sound filtering ability is put to good effect in tinnitus masking, a technique that is based on the artificial creation of an *additional* sound that's aimed at reducing the impact of tinnitus noises. This is how it works:

◆ The masking device produces a sound, which although perhaps louder than that of the tinnitus, will be of a kind that the brain finds easier to ignore. Although all kinds of noises can result from tinnitus, the most common ones are fairly high-pitched tones, and these are not only often exceptionally unpleasant but also particularly difficult to ignore. On the other hand, for example, a sound like the gentle gurgling of a fountain is a lot easier to ignore and even when consciously perceived a great deal more pleasant than tinnitus. In practice, what this means is that when someone is receiving an artificially created sound, as he or she learns to ignore this, so the underlying tinnitus may no longer be perceived as clearly as before.

The masking principle can be utilized in several ways, the most common ones including:

 Electronic Devices Worn In or Behind the Ear. Looking essentially like hearing aids, these devices can also form part of or be an addition to a normal hearing aid, if one is required to help with hearing loss. Depending upon the actual device, the wearer may have a great deal of control in choosing or altering the masking sound, altering its volume and fundamental pitch as well as in what frequencies it will be at its loudest. It may take a while for someone to get the full benefit of a masking device as, firstly, the most effective settings have to be found. While audiometry can provide clues as what kind of masking sound is most likely to be helpful in a given case, the user may still have to experiment quite a bit thereafter until the optimum relief is obtained. Secondly, while the masker may be effective in "blanking out" the tinnitus noises, the user is, of course, initially very much aware of the masking sound itself. Although this sound will be one that is easier to ignore, it may still be several weeks or longer before that is achieved.

◆ **Radios, Record Players and so on**. Many tinnitus sufferers have found that merely having a radio, tape or record playing at low volume can be an effective tinnitus masker. Generally, this will work best if the external sounds are fairly monotonous, so-called "easy listening" music working very well for many people. It can also be useful to experiment with the tone controls—or graphic equalizer—of the sound source's amplifier as selecting settings that heighten one or more frequencies in the treble while cutting down in the bass usually makes for more effective masking. In some cases, the greatest masking effect is producing by turning on a radio, deliberately not tuning it into a station. But with the volume turned up quite high, the resultant hissing, crackling sound—which is a mixture of noises at various frequencies—often being an excellent masker.

◆ **Special Tinnitus Masking Audio Tapes.** A number of tapes containing sounds designed to work particularly well for a wide cross-section of tinnitus sufferers have been recorded by experts. Details of where to get these tapes can be obtained from both The Royal National Institute for Deaf People and The British Tinnitus Association (see Sources of Help and Advice--U.K. at the end of this book for their addresses).

Apart from these ways of masking tinnitus, you can also experiment yourself with a variety of sounds. Some of the sounds that tinnitus sufferers have reported as working well for *them* as maskers have been quite surprising, including such as washing machines, the chirping of cage birds, in fact just

about any sound has been credited by one sufferer
or another as being of help in their case.

Masking, of course, will not work for everyone,
but it will do so to a greater or lesser extent for
many. One quick way of establishing whether masking is likely to be of help to you is by trying a very
simple test. This is what you do:

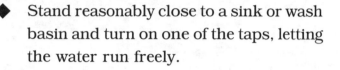

- ◆ Stand reasonably close to a sink or wash
  basin and turn on one of the taps, letting
  the water run freely.

- ◆ Ask yourself whether the sound of the
  running water completely obscures your
  tinnitus. If the water masks the tinnitus,
  then there's every chance that a masker
  will do the same. Should your tinnitus
  still remain clearly audible above the
  sound of the water, then the chances are
  slimmer that a masker will make a great
  deal of difference.

This test, of course, provides only an indication and
even should it suggest that a masker won't help a
lot, it's still worth investigating further in case some
other sort of masking sound will be more effective.

While masking works by providing a more
easily ignored or pleasanter sound than tinnitus,

another way of minimizing the impact of the disorder is by reducing how strongly you react to or are affected by the noises you hear. In the next chapter, we will be looking at different ways of doing exactly that.

Chapter 9
Psychological Aspects of Tinnitus

While medical treatments, hearing aids, masking devices, and the avoidance of those things that make the disorder worse can bring major relief in many cases of tinnitus, it still remains a sad fact that after having tried all these remedies many sufferers will still have problems scvere enough to greatly affect the quality of their life. In these cases, relief may often be found in one or more psychological approaches.

It needs to be pointed out at this stage there is no reason to believe psychological help of any kind will actually reduce tinnitus or make it go away. Such approaches will leave the physical problem which manifests itself as tinnitus totally unchanged, but what they *can* alter is how much the noises affect you and make it easier for you to ignore them, perhaps even to the point where you don't notice them at all, or only rarely so. The rationale for dealing with tinnitus this way is quite simple: If you can't make a problem disappear, the next best thing is to arrange things so it disturbs you as little as possible.

"Psychology," of course, denotes the science concerned with the behavior of man (by the way, animals as well, but that isn't relevant in this context) and this very broad classification encompasses a large number of different schools of thought, some of these based on what at times appear to be conflicting theories and methods. Just how useful psychological approaches are likely to be in tinnitus will vary considerably from patient to patient, but experts generally agree upon the following key points:

◆ While not all tinnitus is directly related to stress, anxiety or depression, the extent to which patients will react to and be affected by their disorder will often be greatly influenced by their state of mind.

◆ An undue level of stress for lengthy periods is often the first stepping stone that leads to other psychological difficulties later. Any chronic disorder, especially one whose symptoms can be as difficult to ignore like those of tinnitus, will in itself almost certainly be a source of considerable additional stress.

◆ While they are separate disorders, there are close links between anxiety and depression, one frequently being the hand maiden preceding the other. The symptoms of almost any ailment—including tinnitus—will appear to be at their worst when the patient is also in an anxious or depressed state, especially if that causes him or her not to make the fullest possible use of such remedies as are available.

◆ It is not uncommon for there to be a vicious circle in operation in which the tinnitus creates anxiety or other allied psychological problems; the heightened anxiety then making the tinnitus seem worse than it is; and this in turn leading to yet further and possibly greater anxiety. If this circle can't be broken by curing the tinnitus, then its overall harmful effect may well be greatly diminished by reducing the anxiety level.

Summing up, this means that anything which addresses the problem of undue stress is likely to pay rich dividends in tinnitus in two quite separate ways:

1) The less stressed you feel, the less bothered you're likely to be by whatever level
of tinnitus you have. Conversely, the
more stressed you are, the greater will
be impact of tinnitus.

2) Because the tinnitus will bother you less
when you're not under undue stress, the
disorder will itself become a lesser
source of stress.

In effect, the two paragraphs directly above describe
the operation of what might be called a "beneficent"
circle where improvement feeds upon improvement, and which is the very opposite of a vicious
one. Looking at it another way, if you've done all you
can to minimize your tinnitus and it's still troubling
you greatly, you may yet achieve a substantial reduction in how you perceive it by reducing your
stress level.

What Exactly is Stress?

In a medical context, stress is normally defined as
any factor that threatens the health of the body or
has an adverse effect on its functioning. However,
psychologists generally prefer a different definition
that states: "Stress is the nonspecific response of

the body to any demand." The key part of this last definition, of course, is the phrase "nonspecific," which identifies in other words, a response that isn't necessary or useful in dealing with the problem at hand. For example, getting agitated about your tinnitus isn't going to help you cope any better with its symptoms, yet that is exactly what happens quite often.

There are many different kinds of tests and psychological inventories aimed at determining whether someone is unduly stressed, but these are likely to be rather superfluous in the case of someone afflicted with severe tinnitus. Generally, it can be safely assumed that anyone in that position is subject to a high level of stress, the cumulative effect of this possibly leading to anxiety.

While there are many ways to reduce stress and/or anxiety, the ones used most commonly when tinnitus is the main problem are either drug treatments or relaxation techniques, or, of course, a combination of both these approaches.

Drug Treatments to Relieve Stress

Whether or not you should take drugs to relieve stress to make it easier to cope with tinnitus is, of course, a question for your doctor, but the way you choose to present your problems may well affect his decision. Drugs that may prescribed include:

◆ **Benzodiazepines.** These drugs—*lorazepam* and *diazepam* are probably the best known and most widely prescribed examples—were first introduced more than 30 years ago and are still considered to be a first line of defense against anxiety symptoms. Although the Committee on Safety of Medicines has recommended that benzodiazepines were to be considered as inappropriate for the treatment of short-term "mild" anxiety, this recommendation has by no means been fully observed by many family doctors.

While these drugs can be highly effective, they do have a high risk of dependence and many patients have had great difficulties in coming off them. There are also some possible side effects, including drowsiness, headaches and vertigo.

◆ **MAOIs**. The initials stand for "monoamine oxidase inhibitors." Used to treat both anxiety and depression, these drugs are particularly effective in treating high levels of stress that culminate in so-called "panic attacks." Great caution, however, must be exercised with these medications because they can interact dangerously with some common foods as well as with other drugs so their use is usually avoided when safer preparations may be equally suitable.

◆ **Antidepressants.** Despite their name, these can be more effective in the treatment of anxiety than drugs meant specifically for that purpose, and they also carry a much lower risk of dependency. On the other hand, antidepressants can be slow in producing results and patients may not persevere with them long enough to gain worthwhile benefits. Additionally, these drugs have been known to create as side effects some of the very symptoms that patients are most concerned about, such as apprehension, insomnia and irritability. Antidepressants have to be used very cautiously in tinnitus because they can in fact make the problem worse.

For additional information about some of these drugs, see the section headed "Drug Treatments for Tinnitus" at the end of Chapter 6 and that headed "Drugs that May Worsen Matters" in Chapter 7.

Relaxation Techniques

While drugs may bring rapid relief from stress and anxiety, this treatment merely reduces the symptoms that an emotional overload may create. Useful though that can be to get someone over a bad patch, it is not an ideal long term solution. On the other hand, relaxation techniques when used properly can be equally effective in combating stress and anxiety, this being accomplished without any risk of side effects or harmful dependence.

There are many different kinds of relaxation methods, but the ones used most commonly to relieve anxiety are all based on the principle that the sought after mental relaxation will come as a by-product of seeking and attaining physical relaxation. This view essentially amounts to saying: "If the body can be brought to a state of deep physical relaxation, then the mind, too, will become relaxed, so dissipating stress and tension." For more sceptical readers, it perhaps need to be added that the idea of using the body to relax the mind—or vice versa—is one whose validity has been proven beyond doubt by countless experimental studies.

For more information about relaxation techniques:

 Ask your family doctor. Many of the more enlightened practices nowadays operate special classes where relaxation techniques are taught to patients who are likely to benefit from them.

 Alternatively, your doctor may refer you to your local hospital where almost certainly relaxation techniques are taught either on a one-to-one basis or in group sessions.

 Check with your local adult education institute for relaxation classes.

 Should none of these approaches yield results, you'll almost certainly find several "do-it-yourself books" on the subject at your local library.

Other Psychologically-Based Approaches

The following stress-reduction techniques are only likely to be available to patients in special Tinnitus

Clinics attached to the Ear, Nose and Throat Departments of larger hospitals. Generally, only patients with severe tinnitus that is considerably aggravated by stress and/or anxiety will be candidates for these treatments which often form part of a research program.

◆ **Biofeedback training.** This technique works by providing the subject with immediate information about a bodily function that normally operates unconsciously. During a biofeedback training session, the patient is connected to a monitoring instrument measuring unconscious body activities, such as blood pressure, pulse rate, body temperature, and muscle tension. The monitoring equipment feeds information about changes in the activities levels to the patient, either through flashing lights, a needle moving on a dial, or a tone whose pitch alters. Usually, after some practice, the patient learns how to exercise a degree of conscious control over the unconscious function being monitored. In tinnitus, the technique has been used with some success to reduce muscular tension, promoting overall relaxation, which leads to lessened perception of the noises. Most commonly, biofeedback is used in conjunction with normal deep relaxation techniques.

◆ **Cognitive-behavioral therapy.** Based on the idea that the way we perceive our environment and ourselves influences our emotions and behavior, cognitive-behavioral therapy seeks to alter these perceptions into more positive ones by changing the way the patient interprets events. For example, someone suffering from anxiety or depression may believe that undesirable events are the result of a failing on his or her part. The therapist will attempt to identify negative attitudes and irrational beliefs, leading the patient to see problems more positively and optimistically, thereby automatically easing anxiety or emotional distress associated with them. If a patient can be brought to see his problem as less troublesome, then it often follows that its symptoms will bother him less.

Psychological approaches also often play a large part in many of the alternative or complementary medicine treatments which are discussed in the next chapter.

Chapter 10
Alternative Medicine Treatments for Tinnitus

Because there is often little that conventional medicine can do in many cases of tinnitus, it is not surprising that many sufferers have sought help from practitioners of so-called alternative or complementary therapies. While it is unlikely that these therapies will be able to address the cause of the tinnitus or cure it, it is a fact that they can at times be of great assistance in altering the patient's perception of the problem and so make it easier to bear. While this is not a cure, it can certainly go a long way towards making the situation more acceptable.

Generally, alternative therapies emphasize a patient's overall well-being instead of concentrating solely on a given ailment. This sort of approach, which normally uses a wide variety of methods to alleviate mental and/or emotional stress, can work very well for some tinnitus sufferers and pay rich dividends in enhanced quality of life.

While the reasons someone afflicted by a chronic health problem may seek help from practitioners of alternative forms of medicine are highly individual, the main ones, according to a recent survey, include:

◆ If there is no definite, clear-cut cause for a disorder and its existence may be linked to emotional states, patients may conclude that alternative treatments with their emphasis on the "whole person" may bring improvements where conventional medicine failed to do so.

◆ Many alternative therapies have a good track record in helping people cope better with all sorts of ongoing health problems, especially those which are chronic or where the severity of the symptoms at any given time is affected by numerous seemingly unconnected factors.

◆ Additionally, alternative therapies—particularly those whose philosophy stresses the power of "mind over matter" —can help a patient comply with some of the health recommendations suggested by their doctor. For example, smoking has been implicated in worsening, if not necessarily, causing tinnitus.

> While it is therefore sensible to give up the habit, this is not always such an easy thing to do. The support provided by some alternative therapies can, however, ease the pangs of withdrawal.

The above are all good reasons why someone with tinnitus that failed to respond to "normal" treatments may want to consider what alternative medicine has to offer. In most instances, it's certainly giving it a try because there is plenty of anecdotal evidence that for some tinnitus sufferers, alternative therapies have made a world of difference.

Having said that in favor of alternative medicine, it should be added it is important to be cautious in choosing a practitioner. While the vast majority of alternative practitioners are highly trained and totally ethical, there is also unfortunately a fringe element whose standards are less than adequate. Because it's not always easy to tell the good from the bad, here are some suggestions that can help you do just that:

◆ If you've decided to enlist the help of an alternative practitioner, ensure that you pick a fully accredited member of a professional body whose standing is recognized.

◆ Although medical doctors aren't meant to recommend alternative practitioners, you may just find that your own family doctor is prepared to do exactly that, even if you have to read somewhat between the lines of what he says. Most general practitioners are nowadays much more open-minded about the benefits that alternative therapies can bring, accepting that disciplines like hypnosis or acupuncture can help some people control stress levels.

◆ Naturally, word-of-mouth recommendations are also extremely useful. Personal endorsements from people whose judgement you respect can be a good guide.

However, no matter how carefully you've chosen your alternative practitioner, it's always a good idea to also consult your doctor beforehand, telling him what you plan to do. Later on, you may also wish to check out with your doctor the safety aspects of any alternative treatments you may be offered.

While there are dozens—if not hundreds—of different alternative therapies to choose from, there are some that, according to reports from patients, are more likely to be helpful in dealing with tinnitus than others. Here are brief details of the main ones that are most likely to deserve consideration:

Homeopathy

Probably the most generally accepted form of alternative medicine, homeopathy is a treatment system devised in the late 1700s by Samuel Hahnemann. Homeopathy is one of the relatively few alternative therapies also used quite frequently by some medically qualified doctors and, under certain circumstances, it can even be available free as part of the National Health Service.

Homeopathy is based on two essential and intertwined principles: first, that "like cures like," that is that the cure for an ailment is often found in whatever brought it on in the first instance; and, secondly, that "less is more," this meaning that small dosages of medication are usually more effective than larger ones. Like many other alternative practitioners, homeopaths also believe that symptoms are signs produced by the body's own attempts to ward off or cure infection or disease.

Homeopathic practitioners maintain that the human body has an in-built capability to cope with and recover from most illnesses and that the healer's primary job is to strengthen the patient's innate ability to heal himself. To aid and stimulate the body's natural mechanisms to accomplish that task, treatment is usually administered as extremely small doses of various medications, normally tablets or liquids prepared from natural substances and originating from a wide variety of herbal, animal, mineral, and metallic sources.

Another of the guiding principles of homeopathy is that of "Minimal Dose," this meaning that ideally the smallest possible amount of the indicated active ingredient should be prescribed, this in practice leading to remedies supplied in a form that is so diluted that often none of the original healing ingredient can still be detected in the final mixture or solution. Naturally, this has led sceptics to question how a medicine can have a therapeutic effect if there is nothing—or at best, very little—left in it of the original "healing" substance? Homeopaths themselves are the first to freely admit that they also don't know why these extremely diluted remedies should have any effect, but point with pride to the vast mountain of clinical evidence that appears to prove beyond doubt that it often does.

Because homeopathic remedies are so diluted, you don't need a prescription to buy them and you can obtain them across the counter in many pharmacies and health stores. While this theoretically makes it possible for a patient to prescribe his own medication, practitioners point out it takes a great deal of skill and experience to choose the correct remedy for a given situation as their diagnostic procedure takes into account not only the nature of the ailment but also the patient as whole. As a result, different remedies may be prescribed for different forms of the same problem.

For example, if you look up tinnitus (incidentally, that heading is cross-referenced to "Noises in the head") in *The Prescriber*, a kind of mini-bible that lists the main homeopathic preparations, you will find that the suggested treatment depends on a number of factors, these including the nature of the sounds heard, such as buzzing. roaring. hissing, tingling, thundering and so on; whether the condition is chronic or not; and whether there is also observable deafness. Additionally, the treatment will also need to be matched to other aspects of the patient's health. With so many possible permutations, choosing the right remedy and dosage is obviously something that requires an expert.

You can get more information about homeopathy from:

The British Homeopathic Association (BHA)
15 Clerkenwell Close
London EC1R 0AA

Tel: 020 7566 7800   Fax: 020 7566 7815
www.trusthomeopathy.org

The Society of Homeopaths
4a Artizan Road
Northampton NN1 4HU
Tel: 015 0462 1400   Fax: 016 0462 2622
www.homeopathy-soh.org
Email: info@homeopathy-soh.org

Acupuncture and Acupressure

One of the most revered of the ancient Oriental medical arts, acupuncture was first widely practiced in China more than 2,000 years ago. The therapy works by using fine needles—or other similar objects—to stimulate specific points on the body so as to create changes in other parts of it. One of the aims of this system is to "rebalance" forces to improve health.

Acupuncturists believe the Chinese philosophy that there is a basic life force—called chi—which is composed of two flows of energy, a positive one known as yin and a negative one called yang. These energy flows course throughout the body along channels known as meridians, and disease and pain, say the practitioners, are the result of an imbalance or an interruption in their normal flow.

Although acupuncture has become one of the better established and widely accepted forms of alternative medicine in the Western world and has a long record of being effective in treating a wide range of disorders, there is a great deal of doubt about whether it can truly make much of a difference in tinnitus, there being little or no objective evidence to demonstrate this. Despite that, there is no question that there are many tinnitus sufferers who most emphatically believe that acupuncture has helped them, this claim being dismissed by most medical researchers who attribute any perceived improvement to a placebo effect.

Acupressure works broadly on the same principles—and can provide similar benefits—as acupuncture. The essential difference between the two approaches is that the various pressure points on the body are massaged by the practitioner's finger or thumb instead of being stimulated by the introduction of needles.

One big advantage of this method is that it is often possible for patients to be taught how to perform this massage for themselves and so be able to continue their treatment on their own, using it as often as required.

Most acupuncturists also offer acupressure, not because it's necessarily any better but because some people just cannot face the idea of having needles stuck into them. Because it's absolutely essential that the needles used in acupuncture be sterile, it's always best to consult a fully qualified practitioner. You can get a list of registered acupuncturists by writing to:

The British Medical Acupuncture Society
12 Marbury House, Higher Whitley
Warrington, Cheshire WA4 4QW
Tel: 019 2573 0727   Fax: 019 2573 0492
www.medical-acupuncture.co.uk
Email: Admin@medical-acupuncture.org.uk

Hypnosis and Hypnotherapy

Of all the alternative therapies used to minimize the effects of tinnitus, hypnosis and hypnotherapy are two of the most successful. The effects of these approaches, which are used both by doctors and alternative practitioners, are well documented and have at times given excellent results in treating tinnitus sufferers whose symptoms had failed to respond to other treatments. Because there is, of course, a great deal of difference between the use of hypnosis by medical doctors and how it may be practiced by someone whose qualifications are more doubtful, it is particularly important that you choose your hypnotherapist with great care.

Both hypnosis and hypnotherapy rely essentially on the power of suggestion, whether this suggestion comes from the therapist or from the patient himself. In fact, there is a school of thought that no one is ever hypnotized by someone else; what invariably happens is that, despite appearances to the contrary, the subject hypnotizes himself, the hypnotist merely providing a conduit for this self-hypnosis. Be that as it may, one extremely valuable aspect of hypnosis is that most patients can be successfully taught to hypnotize themselves and they can then thereafter use the technique on their own whenever needed to further reinforce suggestions received during previous sessions.

A good deal of research has done into the effectiveness of hypnosis in tinnitus and although there are some variations in the findings of different studies, the general conclusions were that for many—perhaps even for most—tinnitus sufferers, hypnosis if administered by a properly trained practitioner could often bring worthwhile benefits, the technique is particularly suitable for reducing the effects of tinnitus that was exacerbated by stress or worry. Experts, however, agree that hypnosis will not actually reduce the tinnitus itself, but will make it appear better as the patient's reaction to his tinnitus is modified, either by making him less aware of the noises or increasing his level of tolerance to them, both of these aims generally achieved by improving his ability to relax and also respond less forcefully to stress.

Despite the claims of some practitioners, not every one is a suitable candidate for hypnosis and there is considerable variation in the degreepeople respond to the technique, some falling almost immediately into a deep trancelike state at the first suggestion while others totally fail to respond. Incidentally, there is no need to attain a deep hypnotic state for hypnosis to work, all that's needed is the lightest of trances. Post-hypnotic suggestions can work extremely well even if the subject's trance is so minimal that he remains totally unaware that he is or has been in an hypnotic state.

One way of trying out hypnosis at little cost and with minimal risk is by buying one or more of the self-hypnosis tapes that are commonly advertised in newspapers and magazines. While these tapes can be most useful, they are, of course, usually aimed at creating generally beneficial effects—such as creating relaxation or improving self-confidence—and not geared specifically to tinnitus. However, many of these tapes can be adapted by the user so that the suggestions they contain become directly relevant to the problem. Incidentally, many hypnotists will provide patients with an individualized tape they can use at home.

Just how successful "taped" hypnosis can be was demonstrated in a study of 32 tinnitus patients: each initially received a one-hour session with a therapist during which post-hypnotic suggestions were implanted and a tape was made, this containing suggestions that the tinnitus noises were gradually becoming less troublesome. For the next month the patients were told to listen to the tape once every day at home. At end of the study, it was found that 22—or just over two thirds—of the patients reported that they were "considerably" less troubled by their tinnitus.

Although many hypnotherapists are medically qualified doctors, many others are not, and you have to decide for yourself whether you want your hypnotherapist also to be a doctor, this generally being advisable. On the other hand, a hypnotherapist who isn't medically qualified may be more experienced and perhaps more approachable. If you believe that hypnosis could help you, you should discuss this first with your doctor and, if he agrees with your point of view, he may be able to suggest a colleague who practices the technique.

Alternatively, you can get more information from:

The British Society of Hypnotherapists (1950)
37 Orbain Road
Fulham, London SW6 7JZ
Tel: 020 7385 1166
www.bsh1950.fsnet.co.uk
Email: sy@bsh1950.fsnet.co.uk

The International Association of Hypno-analysts
P. O. Box 417
Cambridge CB2 1WE, England, U.K.
Tel: 017 6326 1181   Fax: 017 6326 0214
www.hypnoanalysis.com
Email: training@theiah.com

The World Federation of Hypnotherapists (1981)
Incorporating *The British Association of*
    Therapeutical Hypnotists (1951)
3 Clifton Park
Cromer, Norfolk NR27 9BE
Tel: 012 6351 2046

The National Register of Hypnotherapists and
    Psychotherapists
12 Cross Street
Nelson, Lancashire BB9 7EN
Tel: 012 826 99378   Fax: 012 826 98633
www.nrhp.co.uk

The National Council of Psychotherapists and
    Hypnotherapists Register
35 Old Lane
Cobham KT11 1NW
Tel: 014 8328 3592

The Association of Holistic Hypnotherapists
31 Hurst Road
Eastbourne BN21 2PJ
Tel: 013 2372 3454

For more information go to:

www.hypnosis.org.uk

Yoga

Yoga is a very ancient discipline originally developed in the Indian subcontinent. There are many different forms of yoga, but these can be divided into two main categories:

1) Physical exercises—mainly involving stretching the limbs, back and neck, promoting strength and flexibility as well as emphasizing breath control;

and

2) A meditation discipline that aims to help the subject achieve a state of peace and harmony in the inner self through mental control and relaxation.

Of course, both of these aspects of yoga are meant to work together to bring about a "healthy mind in a healthy body." However, the physical exercises can be practiced on their own.

Yoga—although often recommended to their patients by specialists—has not been objectively proven to be able to reduce tinnitus, but there is little doubt that it can help create a state of mind in which the reaction to the noises is reduced, the extent of this reduction being at times so great that some patients have claimed that yoga "cured" their tinnitus.

Yoga also has a proven record as being extremely effective in reducing stress levels, thereby being of likely benefit to many tinnitus sufferers. For those who can spare the considerable time involved in learning them, the meditation techniques, too, have shown they can help reduce the effects of tinnitus.

While nearly all yoga exercises are considered safe for a moderately fit person, there are nevertheless some that create great strain on the back and abdomen and as such should be approached with caution, under the guidance of a competent teacher. Sufferers from glaucoma would also be well advised to avoid any exercises involving holding an upside down position for any length of time. For these reasons, all but the very simplest of yoga exercises should only be undertaken under proper supervision. It's also a good idea to check beforehand with your doctor whether he thinks yoga is a good idea in the circumstances of your particular case.

You can get more information from:

The British Wheel of Yoga (BWY)
25 Jermyn Street
Sleaford, Lincolnshire NG34 7RU
Tel: 015 2930 6851   Fax: 015 2930 3233
www.bwy.org.uk
Email: office@bwy.org.uk

The Yoga for Health Foundation
Ickwell Bury, Northill
Biggleswade, Bedfordshire SG18 9EF
Tel: 017 6762 7271   Fax: 017 6762 7266
www.yogaforhealthfoundation.co.uk
Email: admin@yogaforhealthfoundation.co.uk

Other Alternative Therapies

The three disciplines described above, although part of "alternative medicine," are nevertheless so well established that they are often seen as an adjunct to conventional treatment rather than an alternative to it. There are, however, also several other complementary therapies which have been found to be helpful by at least some tinnitus sufferers. Here are details of some other alternative therapies you may wish to consider.

Naturopathy. Also known as "naturopathic medicine," this broadly-based system combines a wide variety of natural therapeutic and healing techniques under a virtually all-encompassing umbrella. Naturopathy can perhaps be best described as mixture of traditional folk wisdom and modern medicine. The main underlying principle of this therapy is that the root-cause of all disease is the accumulation of waste products and toxins in the human body, this accumulation usually being the result of a life-style that is "deficient."

Like many other alternative practitioners, naturopaths also subscribe to the view that the body has the wisdom and power to heal itself, providing we enhance rather than interfere with this natural process. As far as treatments are concerned, naturopathy relies heavily on herbal preparations and diet management techniques. Treatments offered by a naturopath may include the following: physiotherapy (based on water), ultrasound, heat, or cold, or a combination of these; yoga and breathing exercises; biofeedback techniques; corrective nutrition; as well as some others.

A key aspect of the naturopathic approach is that it relies heavily on the practitioner and patient discussing and agreeing upon what therapies to use. It also emphasizes the promotion of psychological health and the benefits of stress reduction. Although individual patients' experiences vary, many have said it has helped them cope better with tinnitus.

You can get more information from:

*The General Council and Register of
   Naturopaths (GCRN)*

AND

The British Naturopathic Association (BNA)
   Goswell House
   2 Goswell Road
   Street, Somerset BA16 0JG, U.K.
   Tel: 087 0745 6984   Fax: 087 0745 6985
   (For GCRN) www.naturopathy.org.uk
   (For BNA) www.naturopaths.org.uk
   Email: admin@naturopathy.org.uk

Herbalism. Also known as "herbal medicine," herbalism—almost certainly the most ancient of all the systems of medicine—uses plants and their products to prevent and treat disease. In this context it needs to be noted that there is a difference between what the word "herb" means to a botanist—any plant that doesn't have woody fibres and no persistent parts above the ground—and to a herbalist for whom it denotes any plant which is credited with having medicinal value. Accordingly, herbal medicine encompasses the use of any plant as well as any part of it, such as the leaf, stem, seed, root, bark or flower.

Most modern herbalists practice their discipline in keeping with the age-old tradition that decrees that medicines are not just used to treat disease, but also are a way to return the body's balance to its normal state, disease or pain being considered as "abnormal" states. Naturally, this means that a given disorder may not always be treated by the same herbal preparation as deciding what is the right treatment in a given case will also usually be influenced by other factors, these including the patient's general health, disposition, and even personality. Despite this highly individualistic approach to diagnosis and treatment, there are many different pharmacopoeias—that is listings of specific remedies linked to conditions—and some of these have origins dating back as many as 6,000 years ago when the Chinese first started classifying and cataloging herbal cures.

Herbal remedies are offered in a wide variety, the main ones are teas, potions, juices, extracts, bath additives, salves, lotions and ointments.

While there is a great deal to be said in favor of herbalism, a note of caution needs to be sounded: many herbal remedies are just as powerful—and therefore also potentially as toxic if not prescribed or administered correctly—as modern day drugs. This naturally means that these preparations must be handled with extreme care as they can otherwise produce all kinds of undesirable or harmful side effects. It is therefore absolutely essential that herbal remedies be prescribed by and used under the supervision of a suitably qualified medical herbalist.

You can get more information from:

The National Institute of Medical Herbalists
   56 Longbrook Street
   Exeter EX4 6AH, UK
   Tel: 013 9242 6022
   Fax: 013 9249 8963
   www.nimh.org.uk
   Email: nimh@ukexeter.freeserve.co.uk

The General Council and Register of
   Consultant Herbalists
   32 King Edward Road
   Swansea SA1 4LL
   Tel: 017 9265 5886

Aromatherapy. Similar, although more restricted than herbalism, aromatherapy uses "essential oils" derived or extracted from wild or cultivated plants, herbs, fruits, and trees, to restore the body's natural functions and rhythms. The essences are prepared so that they can be used in many different ways, but most commonly as compresses, bath additives, inhalants, or massaging lubricants.

Although there is little conventional medical research to support their claims, aromatherapists maintain the treatments can be useful in controlling tinnitus by reducing anxiety, stress and tension.

Bear in mind, however, that some of the oils used in aromatherapy can in fact be poisonous if used other than in the very smallest quantities and it is therefore vital that this therapy be only administered by a suitably qualified practitioner.

You can get more information from:

International Federation of Aromatherapists (IFA)
182 Chiswick High Road
London W4 1PP
Tel: 020 8742 2605
www.int-fed-aromatherapy.co.uk
Email: i.f.a.@ic24.net

The International Society of Professional Aromatherapists (ISPA)
ISPA House
82 Ashby Road
Hinckley, Leicestershire LE10 1SN
Tel: 014 5563 7987
Fax: 014 5589 0956
www.the-ispa.org

The Tisserand Institute of Holistic Aromatherapy
65 Church Road
Hove, East Sussex BN3 2BD
Tel: 012 7320 6640   Fax: 012 7332 9811
www.tisserand.com

The Register of Qualified Aromatherapists (RQA)
P.O. Box 3431
Danbury, Chelmsford, Essex CM3 4UA
Tel: 012 4522 7957
www.rqa.uk.org

Osteopathy. This is another alternative therapy that has gained great acceptance from the medical profession as a whole. Because of this level of recognition, it may well be that the best way to locate a good local practitioner might well be to ask your doctor to suggest someone.

Developed in 1874 by Andrew Taylor Still, osteopathy has been found to be very effective in the relief of many stress-induced ailments and as such can have a role to play in reducing the reaction to tinnitus in some instances. Based upon the underlying principle that "structure governs function," osteopathy relies mainly on manipulative techniques that are primarily applied to the back and the neck. Once again, however, a note of caution is in order: it has been found in some instances that spinal manipulation can actually make tinnitus worse. It is vital that your osteopath fully understands tinnitus and is aware of what kind of manipulation could lead to problems. Remember that although osteopathy can be helpful, it is also a potentially dangerous form of treatment which—if administered incorrectly by an inexperienced or unqualified practitioner—can end up doing more harm than good. It is therefore essential you find a reputable and skillful therapist.

You can get more information from:

General Osteopathic Council
Osteopathy House
176 Tower Bridge Road
London SE1 3LU
Tel: 020 7357 6655
Fax: 020 7357 0011
www.osteopathy.org.uk

Healing and "Fringe" Therapies

Because the success of alternative therapies often relies greatly upon the link between physical and mental well-being—a link whose importance is nowadays fully accepted by conventional modern medicine—it can be extremely difficult to gauge what can orcan not possibly be helpful for at least some tinnitus sufferers. Even "fringe" disciplines have their staunch supporters who say that these have helped them "accept" their tinnitus and that this acceptance has made the condition less disabling. Here are brief details of the two most commonly encountered "healing therapies":

Healing. There are many different kinds of so-called "healing" techniques, these include, amongst many others, faith healing, laying on of hands, psychic healing, spiritual healing and energy healing.

Healers have, of course, throughout the ages been given credit for "curing" or alleviating all sorts of ailments and diseases, including tinnitus. It, however, needs to be added that there is but little objective medical evidence to substantiate most of these claims. Despite that, as mentioned in the section on hypnosis above, numerous studies have shown how strong the power of suggestion can be and it must therefore be accepted that merely being told "you can no longer hear the noises that trouble you" by someone in whom you have faith or whose "power" you believe in can indeed bring about a positive reaction, albeit it that this effect may all too often be only temporary.

Therapeutic Touch. Like many of the healers, practitioners of therapeutic touch use a laying on of hands technique. This approach is, however, not cloaked in mysticism and is not based on any belief in supernatural forces, but is instead described as depending upon "human energy transfer in the act of healing" and is intended for use by non-psychics.

In Conclusion

Whether any of the alternative medicines described above are likely to be helpful in your case is very much an individual decision that only you can make. Certainly several of these alternative therapies have helped many patients to live more comfortably with tinnitus; however, the success rate of others is a good deal more patchy. Perhaps the single most important question is one you should ask yourself: Do you believe that one of these therapies could help you?

Chapter 11
Self-Help Tips

If you have read this far you should have a good understanding of how your hearing works, the causes of tinnitus, and a general overview of what can be done for the condition.

This section will focus on self-help natural and alternative measures to get relief from tinnitus symptoms. But remember these measures are not intended as a substitute for professional health care advice. You should check with your health care provider before trying any of these self-help tips.

If you have any interest at all in natural and alternative therapies you are not alone. In the past year alone, one in three Americans has used an alternative therapy or natural remedy to help cure a health problem.

The public's interest in natural therapies is so strong that the National Institutes of Health created the Office of Alternative Medicine. Presently, about 30 medical schools including Columbia, Stanford and Georgetown offer courses in alternative medicines.

The following natural and alternative self-help tips may offer the kind of relief you've been looking for—but were unable to find in conventional Western medicine.

Yoga Exercises

Increasing circulation of blood to the head has been reported to alleviate tinnitus symptoms. The following yoga exercises may help:

* Sit in a comfortable position.

* Turn your head slowly to the right as far as it will comfortably go—keeping your chin tucked in. Hold this position for a few seconds. Then turn your head slowly to the left as far as it will comfortably go—keeping your chin tucked in. Hold this position for a few seconds.

* Repeat 3 times.

* Tilting your head forward, bring your chin toward your chest and hold for a few seconds. Then tilt your head backward while keeping your chin tucked in and return to the starting position.

* Repeat 3 times.

Tinnitus Relief Using Acupressure

As covered in Chapter 10, acupressure was discovered by the Chinese more than five thousand years ago. The Chinese discovered that pressing on certain points on the body had a beneficial effect on a different specific part of the body. Therapeutic benefits are believed by proponents to result through an "unblocking" of various pathways to specific body areas which restores normal functioning. Gradually, through trial and error, more and more body points were discovered that impacted particular parts of the body. Now this ancient healing art is widely used throughout the world.

Massage the points shown below which relate to tinnitus problems for at least 5 minutes the first day increasing to at least 5 minutes twice a day. Use your thumb using vigorous (but not painful) pressure.

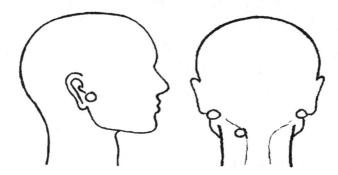

Relaxation Techniques

Relaxation techniques have been of great value to many people especially in reducing stress, lowering blood pressure and improving functioning of the immune system.

Your eyes use up about one-quarter of the nervous energy consumed by your entire body says Dr. Edmund Jacobson of the University of Chicago. Relaxing your eyes can relax your entire body. Try this simple method:

* Lean back and close your eyes.

* Silently say to your eyes "Let go. . .Stop frowning. . . Stop straining. . .Let go."

* Repeat for at least one minute.

Herbal Ear Drops

An all natural formula from Sweden has been reported to relieve the ringing and buzzing sounds of tinnitus. This formula, called Bio Ear, is made with aloe plus the following herbs: ginseng root, bitter orange, dandelion root, myrrh, saffron, senna leaves, camphor rhubarb root, zedoary root, carline thistle root and angelica root. This formula is applied to cotton and placed in the ears.

For more information on this formula call:

Penn Herb Company, Ltd., 800-523-9971
  or visit
www.pennherb.com/pennherb/info/scan56.html

Foot Reflexology

Reflexology is based on the belief that various organs, nerves and glands in your body are connected with certain "reflex areas" on the bottom of your feet. Each of the reflex areas of the feet relate to a specific part of the body. Massaging these reflex areas is believed by proponents to send a surge of stimulation where needed to help clear out "congestion" and help restore normal functioning.

Reflexology techniques can be accomplished practically anyplace. No special equipment or training is needed—and reflexology can be done at home, at the office, in your car, or while watching television. The massage technique is simple to do, natural and safe.

* Sit in a comfortable chair, sofa or on the floor.

* Cross one of your legs over the other, resting the foot on the opposite knee as shown on the next page.

* Massage the foot reflex areas shown below that relate to the ears and the tinnitus condition. Massage for 5 minutes the first day and increase to a least 5 minutes twice a day.

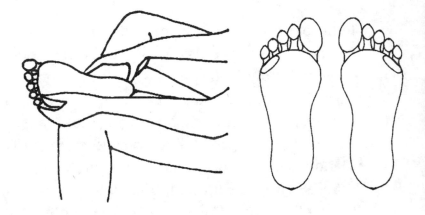

Foods that May Bring Relief

Getting insufficient amounts of specific nutrients in your diet may cause various medical and health problems, including tinnitus. A deficiency of the trace mineral manganese and the B vitamin choline may cause tinnitus symptoms according to *Foods that Heal.*

The recommended daily allowance of manganese is 2.5 to 5 mg. Foods high in manganese include bananas, celery, cereals, green leafy vegetables, beans, nuts and whole grains. If you be-lieve you may not be getting adequate amounts of this essential trace mineral, consider supplement-ing your diet to make sure you are getting the ap-propriate RDA of manganese.

The RDA for choline has not been established, but suggested levels of about 500 mg per day is gen-erally considered adequate for proper body func-tioning. Foods high in choline include fish, beans, organ meats, soybeans and brewers's yeast. If you believe you are not consuming an adequate amount of choline consider supplementing your diet.

Tinnitus Caused by Anemia

Certain types of anemia can cause tinnitus symp-toms. *Foods that Heal* reports that medical doctor Jonathan Wright has reversed tinnitus by supple-menting the diet with vitamin B12 and iron.

Iron deficiency anemia is caused by a shortage of the mineral iron which is required to produce he-moglobin. The shortage of iron can be caused by a variety of factors including a diet lacking in dark green vegetables and organ meats, pregnancy and excessive menstrual flow.

The RDA for iron is between 10 and 18 mg. Foods high in iron include fish, lean meat, beans and whole grains. If you believe you are not getting sufficient amounts of iron in your diet consider supplements.

Pernicious anemia is caused by the body's inability to absorb vitamin B12 in amounts sufficient to produce normal quantities of red blood cells. This can be caused by an inflamed bowel, parasites or small intestine disorders. The RDA of vitamin B12 is 3 mcg. Foods high in vitamin B12 include beef, fish, and dairy products. If you believe you are not getting adequate supplies of vitamin B12 consider supplementing your diet.

Hand Reflexology

Similar to foot reflexology, there are certain "reflex areas" in the hands that are connected to specific organs in the body. Massaging these reflex areas is believed by proponents to send a surge of stimulation where needed to help clear out "congestion" and help restore normal functioning.

Like foot reflexology, hand reflexology can be done almost anywhere—and no special devices or training are required.

It is important to remember when performing the hand reflexology exercises below that your right hand specifically relates to your right ear—and likewise your left hand relates to your left ear. But if you suffer tinnitus in only one ear it may still be a good idea to work on both hands. This may help prevent future problems in the unaffected ear.

* Sit in a comfortable chair and relax.

* Following the illustration below, massage the reflex areas on each hand for about 5 minutes the first day. Starting the second day, massage for at least 5 minutes twice a day.

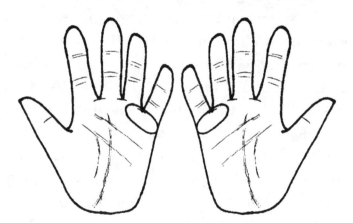

The Herb Ginkgo Biloba for Tinnitus

Chinese herbalists have recommended ginkgo biloba as a valuable nutritional factor for more than 2000 years. Currently, ginkgo products are among Europe's most widely prescribed herbs with sales well over one-half billion dollars a year. Ginkgo biloba is one of the world's oldest trees.Only the leaves of the tree are used in ginkgo products.

Ginkgo has demonstrated significant healing powers in a variety of ailments—including tinnitus. For example, a 13 month preliminary study conducted in Paris showed promising results. Of the 103 chronic tinnitus sufferers involved in the study, all reported improvement after taking the herb. The herb is available at health food stores.

The American Tinnitus Association also reported on a preliminary study in West Germany involving 64 participants. The study reported that the herb ginkgo biloba improved tinnitus in most participants. At this time it is not scientifically known why ginkgo biloba brings relief from tinnitus. While more study is needed to conclusively prove the value of this herb in relieving tinnitus symptoms, it may be worth a try since ginkgo is easy to obtain at most any health food store and it's safe to use and inexpensive.

Yoga Breathing Exercises for Tinnitus

Yoga is an ancient Indian art involving discipline of

the mind and body. Mainly consisting of deep breathing and stretching exercises, yoga is often useful in stress reduction.

Several specific breathing techniques which help clear the inner ear and sinus cavities may be useful for tinnitus sufferers.

Here is how to do the breathing exercise:

* Sit comfortably with your lower back well supported and your head upright and your shoulders back.

* Inhale normally through both nostrils. Then press one nostril closed and exhale through the other open nostril.

* Now inhale again through both nostrils. Then press the other nostril closed and exhale through the open nostril.

* Repeat step 2 and 3, alternating breathing from nostril to nostril. Do this for about 2 to 3 times a day for about five minutes each session. It should take about 2 minutes to "pop" each ear which helps promote cleansing of the ears.

For a more vigorous technique, inhale and exhale out of one nostril at a time simply by alternately pressing one nostril closed.

If your nasal passages are blocked you may be able to unclog them by inhaling through your mouth and gently exhaling through the less blocked nostril until it clears, then repeating for the other side.

Prescription Medication

While prescription medications are not the treatment of choice in this book, one medication deserves special mention because of its apparent effectiveness and safety in relieving tinnitus symptoms. It is called alprazolam—brand name Xanax.

This medication is normally used for anxiety associated with depression. It is also widely used to treat panic disorders. Of all the tranquilizers on the market today alprazolam is the most widely prescribed and probably has the fewest side effects. A double-blind study of persons suffering from tinnitus showed that 76 percent of the participants experienced a reduction in tinnitus symptoms. A reduction was measured by a diminution in tinnitus of at least 40 percent. You'll have to visit your doctor to get a prescription for this medication.

Relief from Sounds

Dr. Deepak Chopra, of Del Mar, California, is a nationally prominent medical doctor who subscribes to alternative treatments to heal health problems.

In his audio tape entitled, "Magical Mind, Magical Body," Dr. Chopra recommends uttering the letter "n" for as long as comfortably possible.

To practice this exercise, sit in a comfortable position and simply utter "n"—almost as if you were humming "nnnnn." Try this about 3 times a day, for several minutes each session. Many people have reported good results using this exercise.

Morning Tinnitus—Some Helpful Suggestions

Some tinnitus sufferers experience a significant increase in tinnitus in the morning—sometimes referred to as the "morning roar." Many tinnitus sufferers have reported getting relief from "morning roar" by sleeping with their head slightly elevated through the use of two or more extra pillows. The specific reason why this alleviates symptoms in some people has not been scientifically established. However, it is believed that elevating the head during sleep may help relieve congestion of blood in the ear canal.

Other cases of "morning roar" may be due to a drop in blood sugar levels while sleeping. Many

·people report relief by consuming sugar the first thing in the morning. This is normally accomplished by putting a tablespoon of sugar in your favorite morning beverage or drinking a small glass of warm water with a tablespoon of sugar. Others get good results from a glass of fresh orange juice.

Chapter 12
Where to Get More Information—U.S. Resources

American Tinnitus Association
1618 Southwest 1st Ave., Portland, OR 97201
Tel: 503-248-9985   Toll Free: 800-634-8978
www.ata.org

The American Tinnitus Association (ATA) is a national organization of self-help groups devoted to providing support for tinnitus sufferers. The ATA offers referrals to professional health care providers in your area who specialize in treating tinnitus. The ATA also publishes a quarterly newsletter and offers a wide array of information on tinnitus.

Free Information from the U.S. Government

You can telephone this little-known service operated by the federal government to get answers and information on any health problem—including tinnitus. The toll-free number is 1-800-336-4797. A specialist is available to answer questions, send you free information or make referrals.

Acupuncture

International College of Acupuncture & Electro-Therapeutics
800 Riverside Dr. (8-I), New York, N.Y. 10032
Tel: 212-781-6262   Fax: 212-923-2279
www.icaet.com

This nonprofit education organization, chartered by the University of the State of New York, promotes research and teaching of safe and effective acupuncture and related treatments including herbal medicine. It works to combine the best of Western and Oriental medicine through international cooperation and shares its findings with the public.

Alternative Medicine

National Assn. for Alternative Medicine (NAAM)
14549 Archwood St., #211, Van Nuys, CA 91405
www.naam-arthritis.lle.org

Provides resource guides of organizations and information for a variety of health conditions.

California Public Safety Academy
www.9-11.com/AltMed/AltOrganizations

This website maintained by the California Public Safety Academy offers lists and links to alternative medicine/alternative organizations.

HealthWorld Online
171 Pier Ave., #160, Santa Monica, CA 90405
www.healthy.net   Email: info@healthy.net

HealthWorld Online offers vast resources in nutrition, fitness, self-care and mind/body approaches to maintaining high-level health. A 24-hour health resource center—a virtual health village—where you can access information, products and services to create your wellness-based lifestyle.

Journal of Alternative and Complementary Medicine
2 Madison Avenue, Larchmont, NY 10538
Tel: 914-834-3100   Fax: 914-834-3688
www.liebertpub.com

The Journal includes observational and analytical reports on treatments outside the realm of allopathic medicine which are gaining interest and warranting research to assess their therapeutic value. This organization publishes a monthly newsletter devoted to alternative and complementary medicine.

National Association for Holistic Aromatherapy (NAHA)
4509 Interlake Ave. N., # 233
Seattle, WA 98103-6773
Tel: 888-ASK-NAHA -or- 206-547-2164
Fax: 206-547-2680
www.naha.org   Email: info@naha.org

This group publishes a quarterly "Aromatherapy Journal." More than 60 aromatic substances exhibit healing properties. When applied to the skin these substances can aid healing. When inhaled proponents believe they trigger a reaction in the brain which can achieve therapeutic effects.

> *National Center for Complementary and Alternative Medicine*
> P.O. Box 7923, Gaithersburg, MD 20898
> Toll Free: 1-888-644-6226
> www.nccam.nih.gov   Email: info@nccam.nih.gov

Biofeedback

> *Association for Applied Psychophysiology & Biofeedback (AAPB)*
> 10200 West 44th Avenue, Suite 304
> Wheat Ridge, CO 80033-2840
> Tel: 303-422-8436   Fax: 303-422-8894
> www.aapb.org   Email: aapb@resourcenter.com

AAPB pursues continuing study in biofeedback. It has over 2000 members in most states. It can provide referrals to qualified professionals in your area.

Chelation Therapy

> *The American College for Advancement in Medicine*
> 23121 Verdugo Dr., #204, Laguna Hills, CA 92653
> 1-800-LEAD-OUT   www.acam.org

Free information on chelation therapy explaining the health benefits, cost and insurance coverage is available upon request.

Chelation therapy was developed to remove heavy metals—like lead and mercury—from the body. In a more controversial application, chelation is now some times used as a means for clearing other kinds of deposits from the arteries, removing obstructions and improving blood circulation.

Colds and Flu

American Academy of Otolaryngology
One Prince Street, Alexandria, VA 22314-3357
Tel: 703-836-4444   www.entnet.org

Provides a variety of free information on colds, flu and topics relating to the ears. Some of the publications available include material on earwax, TMJ and tinnitus.

Food Allergies

Allergy Alert
P.O. Box 31065, Seattle, WA 98103
206-547-1814   Fax: 206-547-7696
www.arxc.com/rockwell/letter.htm

Issues a self-help newsletter on latest food allergies research, cooking tips and proper diet information.

Healing Centers

Body Mind Spirit Directory
w3.one.net/~source/

An online source that provides a comprehensive list of practitioners and products that are natural, holistic, metaphysical, spiritual, or healing related. Use this national directory to find links to centers and associations providing holistic health, healing, spirituality and metaphysical services.

Hearing Problems

Self Help for Hard of Hearing People, Inc. (SHHH)
7910 Woodmont Ave., #1200 Bethesda, MD 20814
Tel: 301-657-2248   Fax: 301-913-9413
www.shhh.org

Provides information on hearing loss and tinnitus problems. Also publishes a bi-monthly newsletter.

National Association for Hearing and Speech Action (NAHSA)
10801 Rockville Pike, Rockville, MD 20852

The association provides information and referrals to hearing impaired people. A number of helpful publications are available.

Herbalism

American Botanical Council (ABC)
P.O. Box 144345, Austin, TX 78714-4345
Tel: 512-926-4900   Fax: 512-926-2345
www.herbalgram.org

The Council conducts research and education supporting herbal folk remedies, teas and other herb-based products. It publishes a quarterly newsletter.

American Herbal Products Association (AHPA)
8484 Georgia Ave., #370, Silver Spring, MD 20910
Tel: 301-588-1171   Fax: 301-588-1174
www.ahpa.org

This organization promotes the responsible commerce of products which contain herbs and which are used to enhance health and quality of life. Their *Botanical Safety Handbook* contains safety data in an easy-to-use classification system for more than 600 commonly sold herbs.

Medical Herbalism
www.medherb.com
This site provides links to medical information and to many resources relevant to medicinal herbs or herbalism practiced in a clinical setting. Includes book reviews, newsletters, history, nutrition, reference sources and adverse effects.

211

Homeopathy

National Center for Homeopathy
801 North Fairfax St., #306, Alexandria, VA 22314
Tel: 877-624-0613 or 703-548-7790
Fax: 703-548-7792   www.homeopathic.org

A non-profit membership organization dedicated to making homeopathy accessible to the public. Their mission is to promote health through homeopathy. Their magazine "Homeopathy Today" contains up-to-date news, tips, short articles and a calendar of events. Their library is one of the largest collections of homeopathic literature in the U.S.

Hypnosis

Academy of Scientific Hypnotherapy
P.O. Box 12041, San Diego, CA 92112-3041
Tel: 619-427-6225

The academy acts as a clearinghouse for information and makes referrals to local hypnotherapists in your area.

The National Society of Hypnotherapists
1833 W. Charleston Blvd., Las Vegas, NV 89102
Tel: 702-384-4420
www.wel.net/katherine/2/nsh.html

Publishes a monthly newsletter on new developments in hypnotherapy and makes referrals to qualified hypnotherapists in your area.

Naturopathy

The American Association of Naturopathic Physicians (AANP)
8201 Greensboro Dr., #300, McLean, VA 22102
Tel: 703-610-9037   Toll Free: 877-969-2267
Fax: 703-610-9005   www.naturopathic.org

Naturopaths are trained as specialists in the use of natural therapeutics and restoring overall health. Where required, they must pass a state licensing examination. Naturopathic physicians cooperate with all other branches of medical science referring patients to other practitioners for diagnosis or treatment when appropriate. Naturopathic medicine blends centuries-old natural, non-toxic therapies with current advances in the study of health and human systems, covering all aspects of family health. Naturopathic medicine concentrates on whole-patient wellness and attempts to find the underlying cause of the patient's condition rather than focusing solely on symptomatic treatment.

Nutrition and Diet

Certification Board for Nutrition Specialists (CBNS)
300 S. Duncan Ave., #225, Clearwater, FL 33755
Tel: 727-446-6086   Fax: 727-446-6202
www.cert-nutrition.org

This board helps establish standards and certifies those who are able to pass an examination. The board can provide a list of qualified professional nutritionists in your area. Their website also provides links to the American College of Nutrition and the college's bimonthly publication, *Journal of the American College of Nutrition*. For additional links: www.eatright.org/healthorg/html

Self-Help Groups

American Self-Help Clearing House
50 Morris Avenue, Denville, NJ 07834
www.mentalhelp.net/selfhelp

This organization provides assistance in finding national and local self-help groups. It also publishes a directory of self-help groups nationwide.

New Treatment Option

California Tinnitus & Hyperacusis Therapy Center
6505 Alvarado Road, #104
San Diego, CA 92120
Tel: 619-583-6612
www.californiatinnitus.com
Email: rjolsson@rjollson.com

Appendix
Sources of Help and Advice—U.K.

You can get further information and advice about many aspects of tinnitus from the following:

The RNID Tinnitus Helpline, phone 0345 090210 (both voice and Minicom). Open Mondays to Fridays from 10 a.m. to 3 p.m. Note that calling this number will only cost you the same as a local call, no matter where in the country you're phoning from.

This helpline is operated by The Royal National Institute for Deaf People and will try to answer any and all enquiries about tinnitus. You can also get information packs and fact sheets from them, and these are free, although a stamped, self-addressed envelope would be appreciated.

The helpline, which is currently operated by two full time workers and a team of volunteers, was opened in 1990 and has handled more than 30,000 calls, or about 25 a day on the average. Says Kathie Price, who manages the project: "The average call lasts about 13 minutes. Of course, there are no 'average' people—and behind this statistic lies a range of enquiries and difficulties. We may receive a quick two minute call where someone wants an information pack or details of their nearest self-help group. The next call might last an hour and be from someone who really needs to talk things over and let off steam about their life and difficulties."

The British Tinnitus Association (BTA)
   4th Floor, White Building
   Fitzalan Square, Sheffield S1 2AZ, UK
   Tel: (011 44) 114 279 6600 #
   Fax: (011 44) 114 279 6222 #
   (this is the number to use from the United
      States—including the # symbol)
   www.tinnitus.org.uk

This is the only national charity exclusively devoted to tinnitus and it defines its aims as "the relief and ultimate cure of permanent head noises." Its current activities include:

 Supporting local self-help groups, and helping to set these up.

◆ Providing assistance for tinnitus research.

◆ Seeking greater public recognition of the disorder.

Publishing a quarterly journal—*Quiet*— that provides advice on the relief of tinnitus and also reports on the latest clinical and scientific research.

 Playing a leading part in the international exchange of information between tinnitus associations in many countries.

Further aims of the BTA are detailed in its *Tinnitus Charter 2000* document in which it calls for, amongst other things:

 Greater funding of the Medical Research Council so that tinnitus research can be extended.

◆ The creation of more specialist tinnitus clinics in hospitals.

◆ Greater acceptance of severe tinnitus as a handicap, especially affecting the granting of various Government benefits,

◆ The free and universal provision of ear-worn tinnitus maskers, through the NHS, for sufferers whom this would help.

BTA annual membership costs £5 (overseas £8) and includes a subscription to their quarterly magazine.

> *The Royal National Institute for Deaf People (RNID)*
> 19-23 Featherstone Street
> London EC1Y 8SL
> Freephone: 080 8808 0123   Tel: 020 7296 8000
> Fax: 020 7296 8199
> www.rnid.org.uk
> Email: informationline@rnid.org.uk

The RNID is the largest voluntary organization in Britain representing the needs of deaf, deafened, hard of hearing and deaf and blind people. Its aims include increasing public awareness and understanding of deafness and deaf people, and campaigning to remove prejudice and discrimination by raising issues in the Press and in Parliament.

The Institute also provides a wide range of quality services for deaf people and the professionals who work with them, which will include information, residential care, communications support, training, specialist telephone services and various assisting devices.

The RNID holds a comprehensive stock of books and booklets on deafness tinnitus and you can get a list of these from them.

Local Tinnitus Self-Help Groups

There are currently almost a hundred of these groups in Britain and one of them is almost certainly to be relatively close to where you live. Contact either the British Tinnitus Association or the RNID Tinnitus Helpline (see entries above for addresses and telephone numbers) to find out where your nearest group is based.

The activities of groups depend very much on their size, but they generally have regular meetings, quite often with expert guest speakers, and they, of course, provide a forum where sufferers can exchange ideas and compare experiences. Some of the larger groups publish their own newsletters and/or operate a local tinnitus helpline.

The Internet

If you have access to the Internet—the "information superhighway"—it can provide a great deal of useful information about many aspects of tinnitus.

Particularly worth checking out is the newsgroup "alt.support.tinnitus." Accessed through an Internet newsreader program, this group includes postings from both tinnitus sufferers and professionals. Just what you'll find on a given day will vary considerably, but usually there will be a mix of down-to-earth advice as well as information about the latest research. Naturally, if you have a specific question, you can also post it here and the chances are that you will eventually receive several replies. This is also a good place to make contact with other tinnitus sufferers, this possibly leading to one-to-one contact via e-mail or by ordinary post.

For more general information, a fairly large amount of material about tinnitus can also be downloaded from any of the following sites:

www.bixby.org/faq/tinnitus.html

www.hearusa.com/tinnitus/tinnitus_home.html

www.californiatinnitus.com

tinnitusanswerboard.com

Interesting Medical Sites

Aromatherapy Organisations Council (AOC)
www.aoc.uk.net

Online source for alternative medical groups:
www.britishservices.co.uk/altmed.htm

Medicines Control Agency
www.mca.gov.uk/home.htm

American Dietetic Association
www.eatright.org/healthorg/html

Index

W

X

Y

Z